ICED!

The Illusionary Treatment Option

Gary Reinl

With Foreword
By Dr. Kelly Starrett

Gary Reinl has spent nearly forty years in the sports-medicine field, with diverse experiences ranging from training professional athletes to pioneering the field of strength-building for women during the pregnancy year to developing rehabilitation programs for injured workers.

Additionally, his ground-breaking senior strength-building protocol has now been implemented in more than 1,000 senior living facilities. Gary has authored two previous books, *Making Mama Fit* [Leisure Press, 1983] and the 2007 "fat loss" book *Get Stronger, Feel Younger* [Rodale Press].

Gary lives in Henderson, Nevada, with his wife, Susan. He has two grown children, Mandy and Casey, and three grandchildren, Harper, Hendrick, and Eleuthera.

www.garyreinl.com
www.facebook.com/TheAntiIceMan
Twitter: @TheAntiIceMan

ISBN 978-0-9898319-1-8

Book Edited by Casey Reinl, J.D., M.P.S.
Book design by Crystal Reinl, J.D.
Cover design by Crystal Reinl, J.D.
Cover image © Gary Reinl, 2013

Printed in the United States of America

Acknowledgments

I would like to thank the following people for their sustained help and support:

To my wife, Susan, thank you for always being there and listening to even my craziest of ideas.

To my inner circle – Nicholas DiNubile, M.D., Joe Smith, Leonard Smith, M.D., and Wayne Westcott, Ph.D. – thank you for your perpetual assistance over the past twenty-five years with whatever my obsession de jour!

To Dr. Kelly Starrett, thank you for the encouragement and opportunity to further spread the "iceless" message.

To all of the scientific researchers, thank you for providing the empirical evidence which serves as the foundation for this book.

To all of the members of my "Iceless" network, thank you for your invaluable input.

To my daughter-in-law, Crystal, and son, Casey, thank you for your assistance with this book.

Table of Contents

Foreword

Dr. Kelly Starrett, DPT

There have been select few seminal moments in the greater arc of my professional life that have led me to confront the limits of my thinking and by extension, my abilities as a clinician. Let me be very clear: meeting Gary Reinl is on this short list.

I should elaborate that while I have come to greatly appreciate Gary as a friend and mentor, I have had to resolve quite a bit of personal and professional cognitive dissonance on his account. What? Some "foundational" clinical practice I have been taught, and have been espousing, and following for as long as I can remember is in error? Does this mean I'm wrong? Have I limited the healing of my patients? What else am I wrong about? How do I know what I know? Oh, and by the way Kelly, if you know it's wrong, and your clinical experience is refuting what you thought you knew, shouldn't you also inform your friends and colleagues? What an intellectual mess.

It was a mess. Until I recalled that central tenet upon which all good clinical and research practice is built. Namely, test and retest. Theory is good, but to talk of bulls is not the same thing as to be in the bullring. Validation is built on observable, measurable, repeatable phenomena. In hindsight, I would have paid a high price to have the conversation with that first athlete recorded. A good coach friend had just torn his ACL playing pick-up basketball with some of his young baseball players. I looked him straight in the eye and said, "There is this new technology we are going to leverage to get you back to one-hundred percent." Of course he was very interested. When I told him that this technology was *not icing,* you can imagine his initial confusion! But, when twenty-four hours later he had no pain and no swelling, he was convinced. His physician put the quality of his healing in the top one percent he'd ever seen.

Great. I had an N of one. What next? Test, retest. Oh, and I started to talk about the ice omission with friends and colleagues. Have you heard of this? Does this make sense? Am I crazy? Try it. And we had tools. Manage swelling? No problem. What we found is that we were ahead of protocols. We weren't managing problems of tissue healing, pain inhibition, and protection. Swollen ankle after a sprain? We were getting athletes to play in record times – pain-free – with no compensation. Military athletes in austere environments were operational faster. Relief workers in Haiti walked out on ankles that were grapefruits. The avalanche continued. Quad sets after ACL reconstruction? Why? Athletes weren't loosing neuromuscular control or quad mass.

The no-icing paradigm wasn't easier. On the contrary, along with the patient-athlete we had to work harder. Not because we were making up for something lost, but because, for the first time, were actually taking the clinical steps to optimize the healing process. We believe that we don't just make the world's best athletes but that we make the best athletes in the world better. Not-icing fell into this ethos bucket. We weren't just monitoring healing, we were optimizing healing. We were leveraging the human body's incredible ability to heal itself by not limiting these almost miraculous processes.

I wrote an article for our gym's blog back in 2008 about not taking NSAIDS for soreness after training and how there was a growing concern amongst the orthopedic surgeons for whom I worked about their impact on healing. That was the first time that I was exposed to full-fledged internet hate. "You can have my ibu when you pry it from my cold dead hands!" seemed to be the general sentiment. Now, you'd be hard pressed to find any athlete popping ibu after squatting. I was ready for the internet backlash this time when Gary and I had our first fateful public conversation about icing a little more than fifteen months ago. Reactions were fierce. Attacks were personal. And don't get me wrong. I love ice. A warm margarita is horrible. If I ever have to have a heart surgery, I hope they slow the metabolic activity of my heart with slushy-icy cold water. And here was the deal. People didn't take my word for it. They began to try if for themselves. Test, retest, share! This is the modern model.

We find ourselves in the middle of an epoch. We are living in a renaissance of human function and performance. People are beginning to take full responsibility for their nutrition and training. And now, we have begun to see that people are taking responsibility for their personal biology. We have tools that allow us to track heart rate variability, insulin, sleep, recovery, wattage, heart rate, and personal biological markers. The Internet has allowed for the dissemination of these best practices at nearly a geometric rate. People are comfortable with a model based on test/retest. The irony of course, is that we are talking about icing! What happens when your iced tissues warm back up? Your body continues to do the thing it intended to do anyway. Heal itself! We are talking about optimization! Is what we are doing the best thing to do? The question is simple and so are its implications. How do I know what I know? I prove it to myself over and over again. When I have a new piece of data, I test it. Are the results better, same, or worse? Is the phenomenon observable, measurable, and repeatable? We run a gym with thousands of athlete exposures a week and have no ice machine. We run a clinical physio practice with no ice machine.

Guess what? We figured another piece of the puzzle out. Time to tell my friends.

Thanks Gary.

Kelly Starrett, DPT
September 1, 2013

Preface

Have you ever been to the Museum of Questionable Medical Devices? I have. It's located inside the Science Museum of Minnesota in St. Paul.

The moment that I entered the exhibit space, my eyes and mind began to swirl. There are so many intriguing sites that it is exceedingly hard to focus on any one particular thing.

But, even beyond the official attractions, there is spectacular amusement in the reactions of us, the visitors.

I actually often found myself not just marveling at the questionable medical devices, but also observing the other guests as stunned looks frequently adorned their faces. Indeed, everyone seemed to be mentally transporting themselves back in time – the only apparent way to try justifying usage of the devices. However, despite these sincere efforts, most visitors seemed to remain thoroughly befuddled.

As all of us intrigued patrons meandered through the collection, the commentary provided by my fellow visitors was so entertainingly colorful that it became easy to forget the purpose of my visit. But, fortunately, it was even easier to get lost in my own imagination amongst the seemingly fictional displays.

Prior to my visit, I had read everything available about the collection and the original curator, and so, as I walked through, my brain was constantly replaying some of the more bizarre stories attached to each item.

But, for one particular featured device, descriptions could not ever have the impact of a single glimpse.

When I approached this particular display, an older guy was laughing so hard at what his buddy had remarked about the device that his laughter proved contagious for me. I hadn't heard what he said or yet seen what he was looking at, but the laughter was so furious that it was itself the source of hilarity for me.

So, what were they, and eventually I, viewing at this station that was so funny? Well, once I saw the "device," the reason for their amusement became abundantly clear.

It was the "Prostate Gland Warmer."

The makers of this unusual device had claimed that it stimulated the "abdominal brain." They proudly stated that all that users had to do was sit on the heated probe and let it work its magic. The directions did not specify how long users should remain on this wholly uncomfortable piece of machinery, but hopefully the treatments were exceedingly brief!

Then, to the right of those guys stood a dad who was intently measuring something on his son's head. A few steps away, the boy's mother was pretending to write on her hand the measurement numbers that the father was calling out.

So, what exactly were they doing? Well, they were in front of a "phrenology" machine, a medical device that, among other things, purportedly determined personality traits by evaluating subjects' skulls and measuring the size of the bumps on their heads. Interesting, wouldn't you say?

Anyway, in another closeby cluster of patrons, two adults and three pre-teens were wildly shaking their entire bodies, as the boys in the group also pretended to be going to the bathroom. And what that prompted this odd behavior, you wonder?

Well, the "Battle Creek Vibratory Chair" of course!

The chair, which was reportedly painful to sit on and often caused headaches and back pain, violently shook users – by design! But not without purpose of course – the makers claimed that it would stimulate users' bowels. Oh my!

I was thoroughly amused by this entire exhibit, but still wanted to know more. And, well, this way my lucky day. When I inquired about whom at the museum might be able to provide me further information, the attendant told me that one of the original curators was actually on site. After paging him, she confirmed that he was willing to meet with me.

His name was James Satter, and he was a certifiable encyclopedia on the topic. The thoroughly interesting curator spent over an hour telling 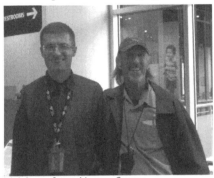 me stories about the collection, the early days of the museum, and even some shocking facts about the early days of the Food & Drug Administration that I had never heard anywhere else.

Then, just before we parted, I asked him if he was aware a more modern "questionable medical device"

With James Satter, Museum Curator

called the ice pack.

He then looked at me and the said, "The ice pack?"

I then asked him if he had ever used one, to which he replied, "Yes."

Like clockwork, I asked him "why?"

He looked at me with wonder in his eyes and said, "I'm not sure, that's just what you do."

After I explained the realities of this illusionary treatment option and added, "If you invented the ice pack today, it would never get cleared by the FDA," I told him to make space in the exhibit area for one more device.

This expert on the topic of questionable medical devices then, with an expression on his face that looked like he had just found a pot of gold, said, "Interesting."

Anyway, with my visit to the Museum through, I began to contemplate what impact this exhibit's crazy collection had on me.

Indeed, this whole scene reminded me of the first time that I went to Muscle Beach in Venice, California. During that visit, I witnessed so many things happening simultaneously all around me that it was truly hard to focus. And, like the museum, this scene represented a vast collection of the entertainingly bizarre.

The nearly-psychedelic diversity of the questionable medical devices triggered my (fond) memories of Muscle Beach's purple-haired people playing the bongos, jugglers on unicycles, body builders lifting weights in the pen, men and women in teeny tiny bikinis on roller blades, three guys on pogo sticks playing follow the leader, break dancers doing their thing right in the middle of the sidewalk, various singers all around, scores of artists displaying their work on blankets near the edge of the walkway, and thousands of people making their way through the space but seemingly never moving.

But, unlike my visit to Muscle Beach – which was just fluffy fun – my visit to Museum of Questionable Medical Devices had undeniably touched off a nerve and ignited my brain.

It proved to be the last straw for any remaining justifications or excuses that I had for why I was not doing my part to inform the public about icing. It was there that I realized that it was unconscionable for me to keep my message contained within my elite network.

From that point forward, I could no longer just gloss over the fact that millions of athletes – as well as tens of millions of others – from all over the country were being deprived of this critical information.

And, seeing this collection up close truly served as the final motivation that I needed to write and publish this groundbreaking book, and then do whatever else was needed to spread the word.

I am not sure what exactly pushed me over the edge, but I am certain that seeing that young family inspecting the "phrenology" machine and imagining all of the parents around the country who just want to help their children in any way that they can – *especially* when they are injured – played a significant role.

The image of parents and kids, young and old, athletes and not, using ice under the false belief that they are solving – or even helping – the problems associated with their sore knees, elbows, and ankles proved to be a powerful catalyst for me.

The thought of this needless suffering millions upon millions of times every year in the U.S. alone was enough to force me fully off of the sidelines. Since that time, I have remained laser-focused and do not plan to blink until my mission is complete.

Indeed, the personal vow that I took when I was leaving the museum still stands as strong as ever – I will not rest until the museum adds one more "questionable medical device" to the curators' collection: the ice pack!

Introduction

Have you ever put ice on an injured part of your body?

If so, do you think that it helped?

It is hard to tell, isn't it?

Your injured spot likely felt colder and maybe even a little numb, but could you tell if there was less swelling?

Were you able to determine if you prevented further damage? Did you heal faster?

Here's the reality: most people simply cannot tell if getting "iced" helped or not, or worse, whether it actually caused additional damage.

And, ironically, it is probably this very uncertainty that has allowed this illusionary "treatment" option to become – and ultimately remain – so popular.

But, with that said, I am not "most people," and I *do* know how to qualify the effects of icing.

Indeed, during the past ten years I have been involved – either directly or indirectly – with the treatment of many hundreds of professional and world-class athletes, have read hundreds of scientific articles on the topics of injury prevention and/or recovery, and conducted over 300 related educational meetings involving more than 1,000 licensed professionals – including athletic trainers, physicians, physical therapists, and occupational therapists – and was ultimately able to tie many previously disparate pieces of critically important information together.

Then, with these findings in hand, I proceeded to personally present this information to the current head athletic trainers of nearly every National Football League (NFL), Major League Baseball (MLB), National Basketball (NBA), and National Hockey League (NHL) team, as well as the assistant trainers for most of these teams.

And, just to give an idea of how eye-opening this highly-credible information was, it is noteworthy to mention that the vast majority of these meetings were held in the teams' private training rooms.

I have also shared this same information with scores of other professional and world-class athletes and their trainers and/or sports-medicine physicians. And, perhaps most interestingly, virtually all of the above noted individuals acknowledge that I have organized and simplified this information in such a way that there was no real reason to debate me.

So, here's the deal: when I first met each of these trainers, physicians, and athletes, nearly all of them frequently used lots of ice. Now, nearly all of them use far less ice than before I met them, and some have even reduced their usage to almost zero.

While not yet complete, few would argue that my reporting and corresponding explanations did a great deal to initiate this industry-wide paradigm shift.

Further, as of yet, no one has ever disagreed that – given my knowledge, experience, and ongoing direct interaction with professional trainers and athletes – I am *uniquely* qualified to debunk the "facts" that have persuaded so many to embrace this so-called "treatment option."

You may be wondering which "facts" that I am speaking of. Well, let's begin with the scientific literature.

After forty years of widespread use, there is *no* peer-reviewed, indisputable published evidence (indexed on PubMed) that the use of ice improves the recovery process.

None!

In fact, several studies actually conclude the exact *opposite*.

I will go into detail with regards to these findings later, but here is a good example to provide you with a taste of the proof that I am talking about. The following is the closing statement from the most recent such article:

"These data suggest that topical cooling, a commonly used clinical intervention, appears to not improve but rather delay recovery from eccentric exercise-induced muscle damage."

This statement appeared in a 2013 Journal of Strength and Conditioning Research (JSCR) article entitled, *"Topical cooling (icing) delays recovery from eccentric exercise-induced muscle damage."*

Next, let's examine the claim that ice reduces inflammation. This is a critical point for everyone to understand – so much so that I have dedicated nearly all of chapter five of this book to explaining it – but, for now, I will just make a quick point to get you thinking.

Inflammation is phase one of the fundamental life-saving healing process. It is the first part of the universally-recognized three-phase process, which also includes the repair and remodel phases. These are all well-established and long-accepted scientific facts.

Fortunately, icing *does not* permanently affect this process.

It merely *delays* it.

Thus, soon after the ice is removed, the inflammatory process, which, by design, began immediately after the damage occurred, resumes.

Further, many people believe that icing reduces swelling.

Since this is the main reason most injured people use ice, I want to make sure that I do not mince my words here: icing *does not* reduce swelling.

In fact, getting "iced" often *increases* the amount of fluid in the damaged area by creating a backflow from the lymphatic vessels.

These two points with regards to inflammation and swelling are a little hard to believe aren't they?

I understand, I really do.

I distinctly remember when I first realized this. My face – like so many of the professional trainers and athletes that I work with – expressed some mix of confusion and anger towards those who pushed this "option" on the country.

After all, nearly everyone says (or at least thinks), "Put ice on that knee" whenever an athlete is carried off of the field or their child takes a tumble.

Regardless of the facts, in the minds of the misinformed, ice is "it."

The problem is, as you will read in this book, "it" doesn't work and actually harmfully interferes with the body's natural response to damage.

Odd isn't it, that so many people actually (inadvertently) believe that their body's natural – not to mention spectacularly complex –

inflammatory process is a *mistake* and that they therefore need to manipulate and/or artificially regulate it by slapping something cold on the outside of their skin?

Chapter 1

The Big Chill

At long last, Spring had arrived in Somerville, Massachusetts.
A twelve-year-old boy was running to hop a freight train.
But he did not succeed.
Instead, he was thrown into a stone wall.
He was lucky to be alive, but his survival chances were waning.
His arm was severed and completely detached from his body!
Then, the unthinkable occurred.
He picked up his own arm and carried it as he sought help.
However, the arm obviously had no actual further purpose.
Nonetheless, his instincts took over and implored him to bring it.
Eventually, a police ambulance arrived to help him.
He was then rushed to Boston's Massachusetts General Hospital.
Doctors worked furiously and saved his life.
Impressive indeed, but this feat was hardly original.
But what about his arm?
Surely it just became medical waste…

May 23, 1962.

That was the date that marked the inflection point for topical icing, but not in the way that you might think. This wasn't the result of the promotional efforts of any person, company, or group, but instead was the eventual public reaction to a well-publicized "medical miracle."

It was the perfect heartwarming tale of a twelve-year-old boy with a severed arm named Everett Knowles that enabled ice to melt into the cultural fabric of America, and ultimately the world.

That boy's story became headline news and for good reason: for the first time doctors had reattached a limb – thanks to the revolutionary realization of Dr. Ronald Malt and his team that putting the child's arm on ice would preserve the tissue, thereby granting his team the time that they needed to reattach the arm.

And reattach it, they did.

A monumental achievement in any event, but these doctors did it without any special tools or magnifying goggles. The chances for success in this case were slim, but doctors everywhere soon realized that future cases didn't have to face such long odds.

"Put ice on your severed body part – immediately!" they yelled, and ice became the integral ingredient for turning body part reattachment into a routine medical procedure. No longer would such a feat be considered a "miracle." Indeed, in today's world, it is far from it.

To this day, most everyone knows to quickly get that severed finger wrapped in a plastic bag and put on ice so that doctors will be able to reattach it. And, to say that this child's story was merely "big news" would be an enormous understatement.

Yes, like many big events, this was the lead story on every evening news program. But, from the outset, this was also a topic of sustained discussion among Americans.

In the succeeding months, countless follow-up stories continued to feed the public's hunger for this story. It was so big, in fact, that it turned both the boy and the lead doctor, Ronald Malt, into national celebrities.

In fact, for the next twenty years, nearly every time a micro-surgeon successfully completed an even more awe-inspiring "reattachment," the news cycle, as well as the corresponding public conversation and awareness, would start all over again. And, as expected, ice was most often a substantial part of the story.

However, there was one issue with all of this, from a news perspective at least: these procedures were all extremely complicated!

Thus, the explanation of tediously boring details about reattaching bone, muscles, skin, vessels, and nerves was hardly the angle of the story that any reporter wanted to tell.

In short, there was no "WOW factor" ingrained in those details, and worse, those minute particulars did not contain information that lay viewers would be able to parrot and discuss with others.

Such a case is a news director's nightmare: spectacular stories which are too technical for the public to understand and too complicated for them to talk about.

So what was the solution?

Well, every time an involved doctor was interviewed, all that a reporter needed to do was ask, "What's the best way to transport the severed body part to the hospital?"

And, predictably, the doctor would appropriately answer, "Get it in a plastic bag and on ice as quickly as possible."

Now that's a "WOW factor!"

Indeed, ice was now well on its way to seeping everywhere in American society as the catch-all, better-than-nothing approach to all things injury-related. The merits of preserving severed tissue were transferred to "healing" damaged tissue by unthinking people.

In physiological terms, this was a spectacular and unjustified jump, but from a "common sense" perspective, it was a no-brainer (unfortunately for proponents, in more ways than one).

Seriously, consider these lacking elements of the "jump" from severed tissue to damaged tissue.

No study launched this spread.

No facts lent their assistance to the permeation of this view.

No credible group recommended this as necessary.

This popular lore simply became "common knowledge."

Substantiation was not requested, demanded, or even sought – it was just not necessary for such an "obviously" helpful treatment option that everyone was now doing.

This was bought into without much skepticism and applied to such an indiscriminately broad section of ailments, it became uncontainable. All of this speaks to the power of those original stories, yet, unfortunately, speaks little of the actual merits.

Those gripping reports were spectacular ignition points for this icing gospel – which soon also included the still-attached portion of the body part – but in no way justified ice's usage beyond these original narrow recommendations.

In fact, if icing damaged tissue were first introduced in today's rigorous medical research environment, the proposal would not make it past the first round of tests. Essentially, ice has just been "lucky," as it is obviously much harder to undo bad habits than it is to prevent them in the first place.

Indeed, if that were the case and ice was just now being introduced, the public would likely never even hear that they should so much as consider using ice on their swollen ankle.

Why? Because any reasonable study would show (and they do!) that the reason that ice works so well for the still-attached portions of severed body parts is PRECISELY the reason why it should never be used on that swollen ankle!

What do I mean by this? Well, delaying the healing process is *always* the result of icing regardless of the intent.

Thus, icing should only be used when someone *wants* to delay the healing process (e.g. shutting down and sealing off blood flow).

Accordingly, with the healing process on hold, inflammation does not occur and fluid is not brought in, thereby making the reattachment process *much* easier.

The reason icing works for the severed portion of the body part is a bit different, but the general point remains the same. Much like any "meat" that is no longer attached to a "body," rapid rotting and tissue death with ensue absent external action – cue the icing (or freezers)!

Those original "miracle doctors" implored the public to help themselves by delaying further tissue deterioration, essentially to buy the doctors the time that they needed to reattach the body part.

In sum, the doctors knew that they could achieve a *better* result than the body could possibly achieve on its own at this juncture. Indeed, doctors believed that they could enable future usage of the body part – despite the fact that "the body" had already deemed the part lost.

However, in any other setting, such interference would, *likewise*, delay the healing process – an action that is enormously problematic in just about every other instance!

Anyway, since nearly everyone was familiar with the fact that meat (flesh) left out in the sun would spoil in less than a day, but would last a week in the refrigerator and a year in freezer, this message was quickly and effortlessly assimilated into the American popular culture.

Soon, the public (and the media) tweaked the original message, turning it into, "If you get hurt, put ice on it."

It did not seem to matter to anyone that this "minor" alteration had moved ice from a well-established, evidenced-based clinical use (e.g. with regards to severed body parts) to a clinical use that still, to this day, forget about 1962, miserably fails the efficacy test, let alone the "do no harm" test for the treatment of damaged tissue.

Initially at least – from a news director's perspective – all that mattered was that the public was keeping this story alive and that was good news for news.

Although it is unknown who was the first doctor to recommend icing still-attached portions of a severed body part to help facilitate reattachment by preventing the body from shutting down and sealing off the vessels, Dr. Malt was the first to display the merits of putting a severed body part on ice to prevent tissue decay.

However, the identity or precise timing of the first doctor to give the infamous recommendation to treat damaged tissue with ice is curiously unknown.

But one thing is for sure: these recommendations have all merged and become so widely-accepted that millions of doctors, therapists, trainers, and athletes, now routinely put ice on their own injuries and/or advise their patients to put ice on any and every kind of musculoskeletal injury.

And, because of this wild proliferation of acquiescing doctors, the "ice age" had begun.

But my personal career journey during this general timeframe gives a much closer, more detailed understanding of what was actually happening on the ground and how we got to where we are.

My experiences include decades of continuous interactions with literally thousands of different doctors, trainers, and athletes.

From my personal training center with NFL star Franco Harris, to the private jets of Nautilus'® Arthur Jones, to meetings with the medical directors of some of the world's largest corporations (such as Wal-Mart, American Airlines, and Texaco), I spent my career endlessly talking with the best of the best. And, I believe that the way this story unfolds from my view is truly amazing.

I will do my best to give a comprehensive recap of how this

evolution of icing (and devolution of medicine) actually happened. My history is so varied in this regard that I believe I am safe in suggesting that it is unique.

My duel experiences from both the bird's eye as well as street-level view – coupled with a resume so diverse as to include training pro athletes in my gym to becoming the first to systematically weight-train pregnant women, and from developing groundbreaking strength-building protocols for injured workers to creating the first nationally-implemented senior weight-training program (which I referred to as "Sports-Medicine for 95-Year-Olds") – my story makes for a wildly entertaining athletic journey into the history of icing damaged tissue!

Here goes…

The first person to ever tell me to use ice was Pat Croce, PT and he was a true expert. But, his protocol was so crazy that it actually caused me to get cold feet about the whole thing right from the get-go.

Pat – who, by the way, was the best man in my wedding three years prior – would ultimately go on to become a sports-medicine guru. Some even say that he was the first sports physical therapist and that his degree in athletic training was merely secondary. Indeed, he was also the first conditioning coach in the history of the National Hockey League.

Pat later sold his pioneering sports-medicine company for tens of millions of dollars and ultimately owned a respectable piece of the Philadelphia 76ers basketball team. He is also a best-selling author, popular motivational speaker, and entrepreneur extraordinaire. Indeed, in one forum or another, many of you have probably seen Pat completing one of his brilliantly crazy stunts.

I give you this preface about Pat so that you understand exactly who I was dealing with in the below circumstance.

So, why did Pat tell me to use ice?

Well, it was 1978 and he had recently graduated from PT school. And I, as a dedicated marathon runner, was suffering from a debilitating injury. For reasons that I will likely never know for sure – my doctor had (wrongly) claimed that I had a bone spur – my Achilles tendon was torturing me.

It was a vicious cycle. It would hurt and so I would rest. Then, once it felt better, I would run, and the pain would come roaring back. It was a runner's nightmare.

After thinking about it for a little bit, Pat told me that what I needed was for the tendon to heal in the stretched position. The problem, according to Pat, was that the tendon was healing too short. Thus, every time that it healed, the repaired tissue would tear as soon as I ran.

He said, "You need to get it healed in the stretched position so it doesn't tear anymore."

This made sense to me, but his suggestion seemed to suffer from a paradoxical dilemma: when it was hurt, it was far too painful to stretch and when it was healed, stretching it necessarily meant tearing it, which was even *more* painful than trying to stretch the tendon when it was already torn.

With a desperate look adorning my face, I looked at Pat and said, "What do I do?"

I remember his response like it was a minute ago, with the completely insane look on his face that I and many others had grown to love.

He said, "I know what to do, but you won't do it."

I said, "Tell me, I'll do it!"

With that, Pat laid out the plan, "Put your foot in a bucket of ice until the horrific burning pain passes and you no longer feel anything below your ankle. Then, while your foot is literally frozen numb, do the following stretches."

As he demonstrated each movement, he said, with the kind of intensity you would expect from a seasoned Navy Seal instructor in one of those over-the-top Hollywood B movies, "Hold each fully-stretched position for 60 seconds."

As if that was not bad enough, he then added, "And, do that four times per day, every day, for three weeks."

Well, I listened to him and there is no doubt in my mind – none! – that this still remains the most painful three weeks of my life. However, I am not sure which hurt my foot more each time, the freezing or the subsequent agonizingly painful defrosting process.

But the bottom line was that it worked! And, it did so in remarkable fashion.

I was completely healed at the end of those three weeks and to this day, 35 years and more than 30,000 running miles later, I have NEVER had another problem with that tendon.

But here is the most interesting point. Not once prior to that meeting with Pat had I ever heard or seen anyone even suggest to put ice on damaged tissue.

Now, this is not entirely surprising given that our meeting took place in what was the first hospital-based sports-medicine clinic in the U.S. Indeed, once such clinics proliferated in the years ahead, they laid the groundwork and provided a springboard for icing to (eventually) spread and launch into the mainstream. But, in 1978, both icing and sports-medicine facilities were in their infancy.

Pat had founded the clinic at Haverford Community Hospital in Haverford, Pennsylvania, and, as I said before, he was a true pioneer and far ahead of his time.

Anyway, Pat's application of ice was both brilliant and necessary … but hardly resembled the type of ice usage that would come to dominate in the years ahead.

Although my memory from the Summer of 1962 is a bit fuzzy, I do remember an injury to my leg around that very time. I was a nine-year-old baseball player for my hometown team, and I distinctly remember my coach telling me, "Walk it off … don't sit down it will stiffen up … keep moving it."

I heard similar orders given to myself, teammates, and rivals more than one-hundred times during my childhood athletic career. Not once did I ever hear anyone suggest putting ice on damaged tissue. Indeed, even when I was the starting quarterback on my junior high-school's football team, I never saw anyone iced or heard about anyone icing.

Likewise, during my tenure playing in a top-level baseball league until I was seventeen, I again never saw anyone iced or heard about anyone icing. No one … not even the pitchers!

While I am not sure that the physiological aspects of *why* the body needed to keep moving were fully understood, there sure was a lot of wisdom in those coaches' instinctive words.

Knowing what I know now, I am very grateful to have grown up when I did. Indeed, just five short years ago, I would have said that I and my peers simply endured an un-evolved and comparatively inferior era.

At that time, I would have said – without hesitation – that my children were the lucky ones, and that they were fortunate to have grown up in an era when immediate injury-response was so much better understood.

But, now, I know that the exact opposite was actually the case. And, that, in fact, it is my grandchildren who are the lucky ones, having come both *during* the information age and *after* the icing bust.

Indeed, despite the fact that the early part of my era was marked with sparse knowledge on the general topic, I still feel fortunate to have been spared the icing "advancement," having come of age *before* the dawn of the icing boom.

And, never was this good fortune more apparent than on June 5, 1971.

That was the day that I embarked on the most challenging journey of my life. I was just seventeen years old, but never again would I feel as sore as I did that day – except of course, two days later!

So what did I do? Well, I, along with my buddy Bobby Shimpeno, ran 63.2 miles from Philadelphia, PA to Ocean City, NJ in a single day.

Why in the world would a couple of high school juniors do this, you wonder? Simple: reckless bombast followed by intense reactionary peer pressure.

You see, a couple of our friends completed this very route – on bicycles – to "The Shore" and they were bragging about their seemingly impressive accomplishment.

To quiet their boasting, I made an ill-advised remark, stating that I could, in fact, *run* that very course. Looking back, I am pretty sure that this would qualify under my mature definition of temporary insanity.

Nonetheless, the "movement" was started and quickly made its way around my school. The next thing that I knew, "everyone" wanted to know when I was going to make the attempt.

I was trapped by my classmates in a box of my own making and backing down from the challenge was not an option in my mind. And, to make matter worse, the talk did not die down – AT ALL – thanks in no small part to the relentless instigation from (my good friend!) Pat Croce.

So I set the date of Saturday, June 5.

I had less than five weeks to prepare.

Sure, I was a casual "distance" runner, but not that kind of distance, and so I started furiously training that very night. My preparation consisted of 3-4 hour runs, 4-5 days per week, but, of course, neither Bobby nor I ever really considered exactly how long the actual run would be.

Bobby had volunteered to do it with me, but he had felt that he was in such great shape that he did not require any additional training. Indeed, he was an outstanding three-letter varsity athlete – football, basketball, and baseball – but was not otherwise a runner.

When the day arrived, we both felt confident and our journey began at 6:00 a.m.

The first thirty miles were simple for both of us, which, looking back, was particularly amazing for Bobby, who had, by that point, already completed an ultramarathon distance run with relative ease and without any serious distance training.

But, then the morning sun started to turn up the heat – and that wasn't even close to the biggest of our concerns!

Indeed, much more distressing was our unrelenting thirst and hunger.

We were both running in thoroughly worn *really* "old school" Converse sneakers – hardly ideal for any run, let alone this one. And, we were carrying literally NO supplies and knew nothing about hydration or nourishment ... but the circumstances sure forced us to learn!

We stopped anywhere we could to get water – including front yards, playgrounds, and wherever else that we could find. But, our lacking resources do seem at least a little bit more justifiable when you consider that the run took place more than a decade before the mass introduction of bottled water and nearly two decades before Camelbak® or Clif® shots came into existence!

At about the forty-mile mark, Bobby started to crack.

It was then becoming obvious to me that he was not adequately prepared for this challenge, but I needed him to continue because if he stopped, I would have stopped with him. Indeed, leaving him was simply not an option that I was willing to consider.

After fifty miles, the sun began to set.

Our run was taking far longer that I could ever have imagined, and we were both exhausted and dehydrated. But, amazingly, we were otherwise still very confident. And so we continued on our way.

When the Ocean City Causeway finally came into view, we told each other that we made it.

It was 10:30 p.m. and we had been running for almost seventeen hours. But, looking back, by that point, our movements were more representative of the "survival shuffle" than they were of actual "running."

To meet the challenge, we simply needed to cross the city property line.

However, once at that point, we decided to run it all the way in to the house where we were going to be sleeping. This extra two-mile spurt put us over the 100K mark and into the heart of the Ocean City.

By the time we finally got to the house, it was past 11:00 p.m. and it was time for bed.

The next morning (Sunday) our legs were extremely sore and we did not want to move an inch, let alone try to "walk it off," as our elders would say.

Nonetheless, an older, much more seasoned athlete named Joe Austin implored us to get up and move around, sternly warning us that sitting still would only make it worse.

While we hardly felt that things could get any worse, we nonetheless decided to get up and go for a short walk down to the ocean. Once there, we fell right into the refreshing water.

Then, on Monday morning, it was back to school.

It was my eighteenth birthday, but my excitement over that big event did little to make my legs – which were even sorer than the day before – feel any better.

When we arrived at school, the word had already begun to spread and we were famous for the day.

Coach Bob Umberger walked up to me and said, "Congratulations. I really didn't think it was possible."

He then looked at me as asked, "When do you want that milkshake?"

He had bet me a milkshake that we wouldn't make it.

While we were certainly familiar with each other before that point, within a matter of months Coach Umberger would be training our school's physical fitness team for the National Marine Corps Physical Fitness Championships, where he would become well aware of my athletic capabilities during our many intense training sessions.

Anyway, as he was walking away, he turned back and (predictably) said, "Keep moving those legs, if you don't, they'll tighten up."

Amazingly, over the course of our recovery time, not one person ever recommended that either of us put ice on our legs. None of our coaches, parents, doctors, or teachers – the vast majority of whom had heard about our epic run – not one!

Well, it turned out that their collective wisdom was actually much better than the succeeding generations'. And, based on my many conversations, my personal anecdotal evidence is quite indicative of the experience of nearly all of my peers. Movement was the key and, thus, ice – movement's nemesis – never even entered the general thought process.

Coach Umberger's advice was very helpful following my run, but his wisdom was even more helpful some months later.

You see, early in the fitness training, I suffered a significant elbow injury. It occurred in January of my senior year when I was messing around on the still rings.

I had seen someone on TV doing an "iron cross" and so I decided that I wanted to try it. Having literally no idea how to do it, I simply grabbed the rings, pulled myself up, and started to lower myself into the cross position. While not perfect, I did complete the motion.

However, within a few minutes after I got down, everything around my left elbow was really hurting, my fingers even hurt. It was a painfully stupid decision and was serious enough to affect my position on the team that I had worked so hard to get on.

By this point, I had proven that I was one of the best on the team and Coach Umberger was all over this issue from the outset. He was very concerned about my injury, knowing full well that it could knock me out of the competition. Accordingly, he gave precise directives for me to follow.

His demands seemed simple enough, as he instructed me to stay off of all the gymnastic equipment. But also, he made clear that it was equally important that I keep moving my hand and arm.

Of course, as this competition was about the most important thing to me at that time, I did exactly what I was told to do. Within a week I was back practicing. It did, however, take a bit longer for me to get back to 100%.

To this day, I am grateful for Coach Umberger's advice. At the National Championships, both the team and I individually would go on to do very well. Still today, even as a sixty-year-old, that remains one of the most favorable athletic memories of my entire life.

However, I also understand just how tenuous that situation was. I could just as easily have been sidelined for months, but I was very fortunate to have a coach that understood how the body worked – and healed.

If he had told me to ice my injury and be sure to keep my arm still for a while, I am certain that my healing process would have been badly delayed and that my position on the team would potentially have been compromised.

It pains to me even think about the many athletes – professionals and amateurs alike – who were given ill-informed advice in the years since my personal brush with serious athletic injury.

Indeed, so many of those athletes have been needlessly denied the chance to achieve their own glory simply because they negatively interfered with their body's healing process.

After all, it sometimes does not matter how much hard work that someone has put in if they improperly respond to injury – whether by simply denying their body the movement that it demands, or worse, hindering their body's healing efforts by freezing its gears.

Anyway, the year after I graduated high school, I founded, owned, and operated the seventh Nautilus® gym in the world. I was but twenty years old, but my athletic history, coupled with the burgeoning fitness boom, effectively insulated me from failure.

Further, my gym also had a complete line of equipment from Nautilus Sports Medical Industries. And, while this is now commonplace, this was an exceedingly rare site at the time.

In my effort to succeed, I read everything that I could find on the topics of strength-building and rehabilitation. But I also had a helpful outsider buoying my chances for success.

His name was Ed Farnham and he was the general manager of Nautilus®. The company was still very young and so Ed did all that he could to educate me (as well as others like me) on all things related to strength-building and rehabilitation so that I would use his products to their fullest.

It was a mutually beneficial relationship, as I was exposed to enormously valuable information that I may never have come across on my own, and he needed me to be as competent as possible, simply because my failure would hinder his efforts to sell additional equipment.

He needed to prove that there was a sustainable market demand for such equipment and I was happy to do my part by learning all about that equipment.

After all, truth be told, I was little more than a glorified gym rat who wanted to work out with my buddies all day rather than hold a "real job." But, for me, that desire alone was plenty powerful to serve as sufficient incentive!

Ed would call me almost every day for a comprehensive "check in." He would make sure that I was doing everything from maintaining the equipment to vacuuming the floor and cleaning the bathrooms. But at least once in every conversation, Ed would remind me of something that he deemed critically important.

Sure, he came at this from a product performance and business perspective, but the point nonetheless applied just as well in the physiological context.

After confirming the names of any new potential clients who had come in to try the equipment, Ed would say, "Call them, get them back in tomorrow, and do a light workout."

He would often add, "If you don't, they'll get so sore that they'll never come back. I don't know why, but if they do an easy workout the next day the soreness goes away."

Since I was very familiar with the "walk it off or it will stiffen up" concept and also recognized the affect that these "new" workout machines could have, I never strayed from Ed's leadership. I give substantial credit for the great success of my gym to that early philosophical guidance.

In fact, looking back, I can now see that Ed was so far ahead of the curve that no one could even see him. Not surprisingly, he never once suggested that I provide or recommend putting ice on any of my clients' damaged tissue.

And, to put it lightly, my clients were not the "semi-workout" types. Indeed, far from that; they were nearly unanimous in their deep devotion to being their best. As such, I needed to provide them the best, most current strength-building and rehabilitation methods.

Before long, Nautilus'® flourishing popularity launched my membership to new heights. Their success had become a direct windfall to me and my success had become a direct selling point for them. It was a truly perfect matching.

As I gained experience in the field, both from talking to hundreds of people about their preferences, and from reading all about the topic, I soon found myself with a full "personal training" schedule.

The bulk of my clients were serious high school, college, and professional athletes, coaches, and doctors whom we would retroactively identify as sports-medicine physicians.

And, since sports-medicine therapy centers had not yet been invented, by 1976 many injured athletes, especially those post-op, found their way to my gym. And, this circle was self-reinforcing, as many doctors whom I trained referred their athletic patients to me.

To my knowledge, not one of those patients ever used ice on any damaged tissue, nor did any of their doctors ever recommend that they do. Indeed, (careful) movement was ALWAYS the key to rehabilitation – not stillness, and certainly not the extreme internal "stillness" that results from freezing tissue.

These personalized movement-focused programs would become a critical aspect of my success, as I was constantly working with new athletes suffering from a myriad of injuries. I am certain that I would never have been able to achieve such great results if ice had interfered with the "movement" regimen that I had all of my injured athletes on.

Simply put, failure would have badly harmed my reputation – and fast – especially since I had so many well-known athletes. Indeed, some of them were extremely high-profile figures, such as former Pittsburgh Steelers hall of fame running back Franco Harris, former New York Jets all-pro linebacker Greg Buttle, and numerous Olympic hopefuls.

If I had done anything at that time to hinder their healing processes, the corresponding results would obviously have been comparatively dismal. But, I was lucky enough to have been completely ignorant of the soon to rise icing movement – and so were all of them!

Accordingly, just like my other clients, Greg Buttle was entirely ice-free while training with me. And, like so many of the others, he was not 100% recovered from a past injury.

Greg had a nagging – and seemingly complicated – problem that he was intent on solving. Fortunately, he relied on the knowledge of the day, which was still conducive to the physiological realities of athletic injuries and not yet based on icing lore.

But if that hadn't been the case, and he was instead content to follow the icing-stillness protocol that would come to dominate in the years ahead, I am not at all confident that we could have solved his problem.

So what was wrong with him? Well, when I first started working with him, one of his shoulders was very weak. It was the result of an injury that he had suffered while playing at Penn State University. Rehab efforts had failed him so many times and produced such poor results that he had simply stopped trying to restore his strength.

However, once I was able to build up his trust, he allowed me create a program to strengthen his shoulder. After we would finish his "regular" workout, we would then spend about five minutes working on the shoulder.

Within about two months, his weak shoulder was as strong as his strong shoulder. And, both shoulders were significantly stronger than the "strong" shoulder was before we started.

In fact, one day Greg showed up at my gym. This was nothing out of the ordinary – except that it was in the middle of the week, in the middle of the NFL season.

He proceeded to walk through the front door and right into the middle of the gym.

Once there, he let out a loud roar as he grabbed me and pulled me into his body – leading from the side of his previously weak shoulder!

He then said, "It works! I can now pull guys down that I previously could not with this arm ... before they would just pull away."

I still have the autographed article about my work with Greg in my office; he was a real pleasure to work with.

A similar situation occurred with Franco Harris. Just like my other high-profile athletes, I trained him in private sessions, and thus no one else was able to see his glaring flaw, which, fortunately, we were ultimately able to fix.

Like Greg, he was ice-free and likewise never asked for it even after the most soreness-inducing workouts. Again, this reality only served to make my job easier/possible, as movement – just like Greg – was what Franco needed.

Unlike Greg, however, Franco was not "injured" per se. His problem was that his hamstring muscles were very weak when fully-contracted. I had insisted that he build his strength in that area, as I felt that his intra-muscular strength/weakness ratio was an injury waiting to happen.

Since Franco was already an enormously successful NFL star – at that time had played in five consecutive Pro Bowls – and never had a related problem with his hamstring muscles, he was reflexively reluctant.

And, I could certainly understand why a running back – athletes who heavily rely on the capability of their legs to deliver frequent power bursts – would be hesitant. Nonetheless, I was very happy that he agreed to follow my recommendations despite his reservations.

The first time that I had him attempt to fully contract his hamstring muscles under load, a substantial part of one of his legs turned into one big spasm.

In extreme discomfort, Franco immediately grabbed for it.

I was terrified and could only think to myself, *Oh great, I just caused one of the greatest running backs in NFL history to tear his hamstring.*

Fortunately, I had a good understanding of how to use trigger point release to relax the muscle. I was certainly not an expert in this regard, but my limited knowledge, combined with my unusually strong hands, allowed me to reduce the spasm within a couple of minutes. To my great relief, his muscle was not torn.

However, with that, Franco started to get off that exercise machine.

I then asked him, "What are you doing?"

"I don't think we should do that one ever again," he replied.

To which I said, "Franco, what just happened proves that you must do it again. In fact, if you only wanted to do one exercise, I would pick this one. You are so weak in that contracted position that you simply must fix your imbalance."

To my great surprise and pleasure, the ever-gentlemanly Franco agreed.

He then proceeded to lie back down. This time, I decreased the weight to the lowest settable level and provided manual assistance most of the way. At this time, he was literally unable to produce enough force to hold even that minimal weight in the fully contracted position.

Well, we worked on that issue in many workout sessions and by the time that Franco and I parted company after three pre-seasons of training (1977-79), he was able to hold more weight in the contracted position than nearly everyone else whom I had ever worked with.

The only person that I ever saw lift more weight on that machine was Bobby Reich – a furiously strong guy who I had spent many years training, from his time in high school, through college, and up until his brief stint with the Philadelphia Eagles.

The moral of this story – just like the one with Greg – is that the body requires (controlled) movement to facilitate the healing process, and ice would NEVER have assisted that process with any of my athletes and would often have hurt it.

Looking back, I am amazed when I think about all of the athletes that I trained and all of the painful soreness that we induced – especially with my routine utilization of "negative-only" training.

And yet, despite that so many of these guys were on the cutting edge of athletic training, never once did any of them ever suggest – even in passing – that it was a good idea to ice an injury before, during, or after a workout.

Although many of them were knowledgeable on the topic of rehabilitation, they all seemed to instinctively know that the only appropriate route to take was that of ever-increasing amounts of stress and movement.

And I say this to again reiterate the point about the collective wisdom in the era before the ice gurus pushed their bizarre idea on the public. Yeah, you could rightly call us primitive in some regards, but our ignorance of icing turned out to be a great blessing.

I point this out because, in today's world, I can think of many instances from my gym days where ice would have been heavily utilized. So many of my athletes were injured and so many others endured mind-blowingly intense workouts that induced enormous soreness.

Indeed, my clients' workouts were often far from the ordinary "workout" of today's average gym-goer. The point is that, under the faux wisdom of today, ice would be EVERYWHERE in this particular setting.

Here's a great example of what I mean about the soreness-inducing intensity that was so frequently present in my gym.

For my Olympic hopefuls, I developed a strength-building protocol that we dubbed the "Olympic workout," which was based on Nautilus'® famous West Point and Colorado strength-building experiments.

One day, one of my clients came into my gym. He was a young doctor still in residency named Gary Michelson. At the time he was an unknown in the world of orthopedics (however, I felt that he was on his way to the top).

Indeed, he would go on to become a genius spinal surgeon and billionaire inventor of the most widely-used spinal surgery products in history, enabling millions of patients to enjoy faster, safer, more effective, and less expensive procedures.

Anyway, on this day, Gary brought one of his doctor friends with him. The friend was accustomed to intense free-weight-only workouts and apparently spoke in negative terms about the merits (read: difficulty) of machine-based equipment – a sentiment that was hardly unique in that era and one which I took great pleasure in (frequently) disproving.

Nonetheless, he was interested in personally trying my "Olympic workout." Since I knew Gary to be an extremely strong man, I trusted his judgment that his friend was sufficiently tough to handle my grueling protocol.

Besides, Gary had, on numerous occasions, intently watched me take my Olympic hopefuls though the workout, and thus was well-aware of its intensity.

I proceeded to tell both of them that I did not recommend such an intense workout for someone not accustomed to enduring such trauma, especially for someone who had never used the equipment before.

Realizing that Gary's friend was unlikely to back off, I then warned them that brutal soreness was certain to follow – if somehow completion was even possible for him – and that light workouts for several consecutive days would be a necessity.

They both laughed as they agreed to my terms, with Gary's friend remaining undeterred in his desire to tackle this epic workout.

I then obliged to his wishes and we began.

After taking him through only about half of the "Olympic Workout" – and at far less than half of the normal intensity – his face turned ash white and dark circles appeared under his eyes.

I had seen that look many times before and I immediately knew that he was in trouble.

Accordingly, I strongly suggested that he stop and I told both Gary and his suffering friend that I was not willing to take him any further. Somewhat surprisingly, they were *both* very disappointed and Gary asked if he could usher his friend though the rest of the workout.

While hesitant, I agreed, but only because they were both doctors and both very experienced weight-lifters. But, as you can probably imagine, I never for one second took my eyes off of them.

When he finished, he looked bad. Sure, he was a very disciplined, strong, and tough man, but he still looked really bad.

Soon, he recovered enough to thank me and they left.

But that was far from the end of the story.

That night, Gary's friend nearly died.

Indeed, his saving grace was the fact that both he and Gary were doctors. They knew enough to realize that he was in need urgent medical care and could not possibly wait until the morning.

So what was wrong? Well, he suffered from a condition called rhabdomyolysis. In lay terms, his muscles were literally crushed. He was on interveneous feeding for several days, but did ultimately make a full recovery.

And, believe it or not, this event actually *increased* my business, as scores of other "tough guys" heard about this episode and wanted a piece of the "action."

In sum, despite the fierce intensity of my customized workouts and the enormous amounts of damaged tissue that resulted from them, nobody ever used ice and I cannot think of any instance where ice would have helped.

With that said, I am certainly no prophet. I was merely lucky to have existed in a time when that was just "how it was."

I would not discover until many years later that we were (inadvertently) 100% correct in our response and that using ice in any of these situations would only have served to make matters worse – and, in some instances, much worse.

And, contrary to the current popular belief, the extreme severity of the tissue damage that so frequently resulted from these intense workouts actually made this fact even MORE so the case.

Indeed, in many of these instances the tissue damage was so severe that delaying the inflammatory response and decreasing the desperately needed circulation with ice would have been enormously problematic.

But, make no mistake; if anyone had ever asked for ice, I am sure that I would have provided it without hesitation. However, the fact that no one – other than Pat Croce, whose remedy had absolutely nothing to do with "treating" damaged tissue – ever asked for ice in the seven-plus years that I owned the gym, is truly amazing by today's norms.

In fact, at the time that I sold my gym in 1980, I had spent the vast majority of my years in business with an utterly packed schedule, so much so that I honestly and literally often did not eat, drink, sit, or even go to the bathroom during what usually extended to ten-hour-plus days, five to six days per week.

This circumstance actually became so well-known among my clients that they would frequently joke about the fact that I would simply ignore normal bodily functions, usually considered to be of utmost necessity.

Anyway, that was an awful lot of people to be fully and completely ignorant of ice!

And, even outside of my gym during this time I never met a single person who ever used or recommended icing an injury, nor did I ever see any of the thousands of runners that I had been amongst during numerous marathons and other races icing anything!

It really says something that even today, with all of my experience with ice – including thousands of ice-related conversations with doctors, trainers, therapists, and athletes in a wide variety of settings – that I cannot think of a single instance when ice would have been a good idea for one of my clients.

Interestingly, this was the case even as I – and most everyone else that I knew – was well aware of the need to use ice to preserve accidently severed body parts. It was just inherently understood that preserving tissue so that it would be easier to reattach was fundamentally different than "treating" damaged tissue.

Anyway, from 1981-84, I directed the largest, most publicized exercise-during-the-pregnancy-year study in history. As you probably expect, most of the patients – all pregnant (or recently pregnant) women – had musculoskeletal injuries and pain. Swelling and chronically sore/tired muscles were the norm.

While this sounded absolutely crazy at the time, I literally designed the program around the sports-medicine model, which was then just beginning to emerge. I was simply applying what I had learned from all of my years training athletes with similar "injuries."

And surprise! Not a single one of the countless doctors that referred women into the program ever recommended that any of their patients ice their damaged tissue. And, unlike the majority of my clients from the gym days, who were often athletes and gym rats, these doctors were obviously medically educated.

Simply put: ignorance was NOT the reason that they did not recommend ice.

Instead, generally speaking, it was their understanding of the body's basic physiological properties and their reliance on fact-based medicine. Remember, just as is the case today, there was no scientific proof regarding the merits of icing, and doctors did not tend to base their remedies on unsubstantiated claims.

As such, since the facts have not changed one iota since that time

– unless you count mounting proof that icing DOES NOT work – the only plausible explanation that I can think of is that the ice gurus just hadn't yet figured out how to convince the therapy world that icing was a viable remedy.

Additionally, not a single woman ever asked me or any member of my staff for ice or reported using ice. Further, you must understand that I was not just some distant director of this study. Indeed, throughout this time I controlled nearly every painstaking aspect of the complex operation.

As such, I came in contact with many, many different influential players in the therapy world. In fact, I did so much with this effort that I ultimately wrote a book about this study in 1983 called *Making Mama Fit.*

My point is that I experienced all of this first-hand and learned from some of the best minds in the industry at the end of the "iceless" era.

To this day, those arguments for not using ice make perfect physiological sense, and today's prevailing wisdom remains wholly unscientific and, quite frankly, silly.

I can just imagine a visitor from Mars coming down and hearing both sides clearly articulated in the same context and at the same point in history (now). I'd happily bet that they would not take damaged-tissue icing protocols back home with them.

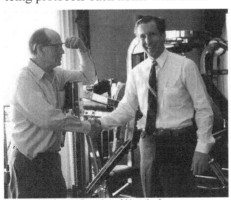
With Arthur Jones, Founder of Nautilus®

Anyway, during those same general years, I took all incoming calls to Nautilus®, both domestically and internationally, that related to exercise during the pregnancy year. Most of these calls were from physicians and therapists, and, you guessed it, I never had a single conversation about ice. Not even a passing comment!

And believe me, those conversations were often right at the cutting edge of medicine – hardly a position that icing could ever have claimed to occupy, especially by that point in history. Indeed, it was not because of a lack of knowledge or enlightenment that our clients did not ever bring it up – it was because they did not find it at all relevant.

During those same general years, I also opened eight centers around the county that provided physical therapy services for women during the pregnancy year. I even coined a term to describe my service: *orthostetrics.*

As a result of this effort, I met with and had comprehensive conversations regarding therapy services with at least 200 physicians (including physiatrists, orthopedic surgeons, and obstetricians) involved with related patient care. And, not once did anyone ever suggest using ice prior to 1991 (when it did come up in a few highly-particularized situations regarding pregnant and recently-pregnant athletes).

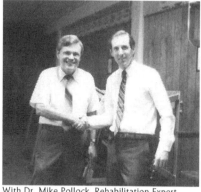

With Dr. Mike Pollock, Rehabilitation Expert

Around this time, I also worked as the host/spokesperson for Nautilus'® spinal rehabilitation medical seminars. Arthur Jones, the company's founder and owner, personally recruited me for this job.

This physician-focused educational program was done in coordination with the University of Florida's Exercise Science Department. Dr. Michael Pollock was the center's director, and when I first met him, he was already a legend in the field of exercise science.

He was not only a past President of the American College of Sports Medicine, he was the national face of cardiac rehabilitation. He literally wrote the rules, the textbooks, and taught the classes. He was a giant in the field of exercise and I learned a great deal from him.

Indeed, despite having died in 1998, Dr. Pollock's work involving spinal rehabilitation is still cutting edge. And I still remember, with great fondness, speaking with him about his research, observing his lab in action, and most importantly, listening to him present to an audience.

My role in these seminars – other than providing relevant information throughout the day – was to simply make sure that our guests felt welcome and appreciated. Additionally, I would spend considerable time recruiting spinal rehabilitation doctors and other high-profile individuals from all over the country to attend the seminars.

These single-day seminars lasted about seven hours, but, since surgeons were normally only willing to give up one day, I usually had to arrange to pick them up and get them home in the same day.

No doubt, this was often a logistical puzzle, but it was not quite as hard as it sounds. Why? Well, Arthur always ensured that I had a fleet of corporate jets at my disposal. And boy did we use them! We had them crisscrossing the country in a seemingly never-ending loop – those were the days!

Anyway, since we attracted the best of the best, I spent many days talking with some of the top caregivers in the country. And, as most seminars had only eight to twelve people, the setting was simultaneously synergistic and personal. The very nature of my job demanded that I find out precisely what each seminar attendee was doing in terms of their rehabilitation protocol.

And, let me tell you, these conversations were comprehensive. I had to learn how each of them utilized exercise, rest, heat, ice, ultrasound, drugs, and anything else that they might have found useful in their practice.

All told, between my interactions with Dr. Pollock and his team of researchers and the seminar attendees, I met and spoke with over 1,000 experts on the topic of rehabilitation.

That said, I never saw a single person who was connected with Dr. Pollock's research use ice to treat damaged tissue, nor did I ever hear Dr. Pollock make any such related recommendation. Further, very few of the doctors ever recommended ice.

However, most did not necessarily oppose the now-burgeoning use of ice either. Most believed that heat was better; and they would often comment that patients don't like ice but do like heat.

True, very few of the doctors saw any use for ice in their treatment of damaged tissue. But, the general medical response to icing was, no doubt, becoming much more tempered than it had been in years past.

Indeed, by this time, the ice gurus were clearly having an effect on the views of some doctors, even though they were generally still only, at best, ambivalent towards the use of ice. And, since this was not based on any new scientific evidence whatsoever, I can only attribute this change to marketing and the public's correspondingly changing attitudes that doctors were adapting to.

Obviously, they did not see anything new – as there was nothing new to see – and so, I assume that they just figured that ice didn't hurt anything and, as such, was not worth devoting any further thought to. But, before too long, the ice gurus would successfully change the narrative and the ground beneath the doctors would begin to fundamentally shift.

At first, the shift was subtle, but the ice age was arriving. Amazingly (to me at least), no concerted effort was made to reassert the scientific process. And, accordingly, ice would go generally unquestioned on its rise to widespread dominance.

Certainly such a scientifically backwards slide is a rarity in the medical profession, but this whole incident might actually be better described as an anomaly, as the only reason that ice was able to make this unprecedented rise (e.g. without any substantiateable proof) was precisely because most of its rise occurred within the media and the lay public, far *outside* of the medical profession.

So, were all of the forward-thinking, top of the heap individuals that I mentioned in this chapter completely wrong about a basic physiological principle of the human body?

Chapter 2

The Deep Freeze

Soon the draft brought in by the "Big Chill" officially ushered in the "Ice Age."

Simply put, ice was becoming equally commonplace in therapy clinics as it is on our planet's polar regions.

By 1991, when I became the Program Development Director for Continental Medical System – which ultimately became a billion dollar plus physical rehabilitation company with more than forty hospitals – ice had infiltrated everywhere.

While at Continental, I was responsible for several of the company's national programs – including its industrial rehabilitation program, spinal rehabilitation program, and physical therapy program for women during the pregnancy year. Altogether, there were about fifty different program sites around the country.

And, by this time, every single one of these sites provided ice as needed to their patients. The ice gurus were now successfully selling their blind faith protocols. And it was compelling, I must admit, as I too agreed without hesitation. It was simply "believed" that *ice was nice.*

Around this same time, I started noticing that the deep freeze had made its way all the way down to parents (me included, I had a five-year-old at the time) and pee-wee coaches, who were now often pushing ice as the go-to treatment option for all things injury-related. Indeed, we were all heading for the iceberg.

While commonplace now, it was really something to see the rapid change at sporting events, where, suddenly, *someone* always now seemed to have some form of ice – just in case.

If Billy twisted his knee or Mary pulled her hamstring, you could count on someone yelling, "Put ice on it!"

And it really didn't matter what had happened or what the nature of the injury was; if something was hurt, ice was the fix. It was the foolproof method that *any* (unthinking) person could give.

But this rapid transition was actually pretty easy to predict in hindsight. As ice made its way to therapy centers, the word quickly got out. And, since ice is easy to use, inexpensive, readily available, and, unlike most every other injury response method, can be administered by anyone – as no special training or certification is needed – it was able to rapidly spread.

To me, as well as many millions of others, this seemed completely harmless and most people seemed to believe that it helped – or at least allowed them to *feel* like we were helping.

Three years later, when I became the General Manager of the Medical Division for Nautilus International, ice was simply part of the deal.

My job was selling Nautilus® equipment to hospitals, outpatient physical therapy centers, and corporate wellness centers. And, even though there was considerable disagreement regarding specific protocols, I cannot think of a single person that (publicly) opposed the use of ice in those days.

My next career stop was at NovaCare, another billion-dollar plus therapy company. I had sold them my "Sports-Medicine for 95-Year-Olds" program and, immediately upon purchase, they named me the program's national director.

The program, which I named "Vigor," was the first-ever nationally-franchised strength-building program for mature seniors. Today, more than 1,000 senior-living facilities around the country use my Vigor model.

During my time with Vigor, I worked directly with the entire therapy team at more than one-hundred locations, and accordingly, have firsthand knowledge of their therapy protocols.

Interestingly, the use of ice with these mature seniors was actually quite rare – despite the fact that nearly all of them had numerous "icable" maladies.

I am not sure if that was due to the fact that Medicare no longer recognized ice as a billable service, if the treating therapists and doctors questioned its value (specifically with this population), or whether it was some combination of both.

But, unfortunately, the good news stops there. Despite ice's rare usage in this one particular setting, nearly every single one of NovaCare's 600+ outpatient division centers still *frequently* used ice at this time.

By 2000, the tide was officially turning back away from ice, in certain settings at least. For example, while ice remained very popular with the public and most professional athletes, ice's usage in the outpatient clinical setting was on the dramatic decline.

And what ushered in this change? Well, a force much more powerful than cold hard ice: cold hard cash.

You see, insurance companies had stopped paying for ice treatments, and the vast majority of the pubic balked at the idea of self-paying for a treatment that they could just as easily do at home for free. Thus, it quickly stopped being "necessary" in this setting.

Anyway, while I left NovaCare many years ago now, I have remained active in this industry throughout the years since. I actually still have consulting agreements with several therapy companies – including NovaCare's new parent company, Select Medical® (another multi-billion dollar therapy company) – which, combined, own more than 1,000 outpatient centers.

Further, from 2000-2008, I met with the entire therapy teams of more than 400 therapy centers, where I provided education and training regarding an alternative treatment to ice. Thus, needless to say, my cumulative knowledge on this topic, as it relates to the opinions and treatment patterns of outpatient therapists, is not only unique, it is keenly refined.

So then, with ice greatly diminished within this setting, what explains the public's sustained embrace of ice? Well, the internet certainly helps. Search for key words "ice, sports, injury, and recovery," and you will find many thousands of articles and blogs packed with advice.

Interestingly, however, if you closely review the material, the same (incorrect) information is often recycled in large majorities of them. Beyond that, I can attribute it to little more than bad habits being hard to break.

But there is some good news beyond the therapy room. Over the past five years, ice usage by professional athletes has begun to cool.

I know this because I have personally worked with the head trainers of more than eighty NFL, MLB, NBA, and NHL teams. I began focusing on elite athletes in 2006 and now spend more than 95% of my time in that venue.

Indeed, I have personally spoken with nearly every head trainer and most assistant trainers in each of these sports. Granted, professional athletes – as well as the general public – still use more ice than I would ever deem advisable, but that is changing very fast.

Mark my words: the use of ice will soon pass and the change will be ushered in thanks in no small part to professional trainers and athletes heavily influencing the debate. Hopefully this book, if nothing else, serves to dramatically accelerate that process.

If you are wondering why I am so confident about this, the reason is simple. Both the academic and lay press have now begun providing the truth about ice.

This reporting has alerted the public – at least those interested in learning – as well as professional athletes, that they have all been, at best, inadvertently duped.

And, predictably, this has caused a massive shift amongst those early adapters who are now transferring from a blind faith to a fact-based faith system of belief.

Below is a sampling of what I am talking about. Unfortunately, prior to this book, these articles have remained frustratingly disparate for the general populace to collect, absorb, and understand, but now, hopefully this book will change that.

The opening line in a 2012 article that appeared in the British Journal of Sports Medicine entitled, *"Cooling an acute muscle injury: can basic scientific theory translate into the clinical setting?"* said it all.

The devastating (to ice) statement bluntly stated that, *"Ice is commonly used after acute muscle strains but there are no clinical studies of its effectiveness."*

Then, in a May 2013 article in the Journal of Strength and

Conditioning Research/National Strength and Conditioning Association entitled, *"Topical cooling (icing) delays recovery from eccentric exercise-induced muscle damage,"* served to blow the issue out of the (frozen) water.

The final line of that article says, *"These data suggest that topical cooling, a commonly used clinical intervention appears to not improve but rather delay recovery from eccentric exercise-induced muscle damage."*

GAME OVER.

Serious athletes might tolerate ice not being proven effective, but few of them will stand for ice delaying and (potentially) harming their recovery process.

Of course, many of us have (rightfully) grown accustomed to questioning studies, even some peer-reviewed ones such as these two, simply because confliction seems to be so commonplace.

The problem with that here, however, is that there is no conflicting peer-reviewed study anywhere from any time in the last half-century.

Ice has NEVER *proved* to be effective – it was just mindlessly adopted by mostly well-intentioned people who *assumed* that making injury spots cold (and perhaps a little bit numb) helped, as I previously explained.

But this news is actually not all that new. Much to even my surprise, the evidence of the physiologically obvious has actually been piling up for a long time now.

For example, the ice was already undoubtedly beginning to melt more than five years ago.

In a February 2008 article in the Journal of Emergency Medicine entitled, *"Is ice right? Does cryotherapy improve outcome for acute soft tissue injury?"* the closing statement says, *"There is insufficient evidence to suggest that cryotherapy improves clinical outcome in the management of soft tissue injuries."*

Yikes! That is a simply devastating report for a well-established injury response method. Indeed, this would almost certainly be the death knell for an FDA clearance if ice were a regulated tool.

But, stunningly, even these clinical condemnations of icing did not come without prior warning.

Indeed, in January 2004 the American Journal of Sports Medicine put the ice gurus on notice that the ice was about to melt.

Take a look at the conclusion statement from their article entitled,

"The use of ice in the treatment of acute soft-tissue injury: a systematic review of randomized controlled trials."

It reads as follows, *"Many more high-quality trials are needed to provide evidence-based guidelines in the treatment of acute soft-tissue injuries."*

WOW! What a bombshell comment!

If only I had been looking – that would have converted me on the spot. How in the world could the scientific properties of such a well-known treatment option be so grossly unknown after decades of widespread use?!

But, as you probably assumed, that warning went unheeded by, really, almost everyone – including me.

So the Journal of Athletic Training tried to give a more effective warning shot in their September 2004 article entitled, *"Does cryotherapy improve outcomes with soft tissue injury?"*

Their conclusion statement reads as follows:

"Based on the available evidence, cryotherapy seems to be effective in decreasing pain. In comparison with other rehabilitation techniques, the efficacy of cryotherapy has been questioned. The exact effect of cryotherapy on more frequently treated acute injuries (e.g. muscle strains and contusions) has not been fully elucidated.

"Additionally, the low methodologic quality of the available evidence is of concern. Many more high-quality studies are required to create evidence-based guidelines on the use of cryotherapy. These must focus on developing modes, durations, and frequencies of ice application that will optimize outcomes after injury."

So, after all these years, we learned that ice can, sometimes, temporarily decrease pain – that's all that they could prove? Really? That is astounding!

Oh wait, actually, it is not astounding at all. Apparently, basic physiological properties did not just magically change because people ignored them for a few decades.

Anyway, in 2011, the university-based and lay press finally joined in.

This lay news-spreading was first launched by the Cleveland Clinic, when they published an article reporting on the findings of their

Neuroinflammation Research Center entitled, *"Hold the Ice?"*

The article states, *"In response to acute muscle injury, inflammatory cells (called macrophages) within the damaged muscle itself were found to produce a protein called IGF-1, which is required for muscle regeneration."*

The lay version of this – that ice prevents the signal to the two things needed to "clean up the mess and repair the damage" and thereby harms recovery – was picked up by many outlets.

Obviously NO ONE would EVER want to do that – unless they were actually *trying* to delay the healing process, such as is the case when a body part is severed.

The University of Pittsburg Medical Center soon followed suit with their article entitled, *"Effects of ice after exercise,"* where they went straight to the heart of icing.

Their article stated, *"For years, athletes have submerged themselves in ice baths and cold whirlpools to relieve tension and pain associated with sore muscles. However, according to an article published in the Journal of Sports Medicine in January 2012, ice may not be the best treatment for aching muscles — in fact, it could even be detrimental to recovery."*

Not that much more is needed, but I want to give you the full picture of just how poorly ice performs on injured tissue.

In a 2011 study, researchers could prove neither that iced tissue recovered faster nor that the iced tissue was less painful (in the long run).

Yet another lay article, entitled, *"Ice slows down the healing process,"* states that, *"A new research study has suggested that slapping a packet of frozen peas on a black eye or a sprained ankle may prevent it from getting better. For the first time, researchers have found that it could slow down the healing as it prevents the release of a key repair hormone."*

Unfortunately for ice, the results have remained unanimous – and are still growing.

Even the Times of India has gotten in on the feeding frenzy. Their article, entitled, *"The role of inflammation in the healing process"* goes on to talk about the facts about inflammation, which I will explain in detail in chapter five.

They state, *"A clear shift in science is taking inflammation away from being the enemy of health and a condition to be suppressed and/or eliminated to one in which its importance and role is allowed to proceed."*

To me, it's truly amazing that this basic physiological response – which is thoroughly taught to just about every doctor and therapist – is even news all. Further, the fact that it is "breaking news" is just downright scary.

It is not even as though critical thinking is required for this analysis. Just think about inflammation for a moment.

Every qualified person knows that the healing process is *required* and that stopping it is a bad idea. Likewise, all of these people know that inflammation is one of the three phases of this (life-saving) process.

So then, who in the world would ever recommend that ice be used to interrupt any phase of this process?

If you are wondering why the ice gurus have not yet responded, the answer is basic: they are trying to ride this out as long as they can.

Think about it, no matter which side you come from, the facts are the same. And thus, since they are currently in the vast majority, all that could possibly come from responding at this point is the drawing of attention to the minority position.

And, of course, since they (obviously) cannot produce evidence to support their illusionary treatment claims, any attention in that regard is inherently negative.

But even worse than this for the ice gurus is that the "fact-based" evidence actually PROVES the *opposite* of what they claim. Fortunately, for those of us who simply want to optimally recover – this is all welcome news!

Finally, in what I have grown to consider the ice gurus' "last hurrah," they actually tried to seize a high profile incident that, at first, seemed favorable to their position.

They went hard in trying to take advantage of this terrible episode, but, fortunately, their plan miserably backfired. They had tried to call this particular life-saving procedure "cold therapy," when the unequivocal fact was that it had literally nothing to do with ice.

Of course, even *if* this treatment had occurred using ice, it would have done nothing to prove their case – just as was the case with my frozen stretched tendon injury treatment protocol that I explained in the last chapter.

Nonetheless, they knew that, if they could convince everyone that it was ice that saved the day, the pesky fact of the extraordinarily narrow application would most certainly have gotten lost in the shuffle.

So what incident am I referring to? Well, it is one that all of us NFL fans will probably never forget.

The patient was Kevin Everett of the Buffalo Bills.

He had suffered a serious spinal cord injury during the Bills game on September 15, 2007.

The initial report was that the treatment was based on the *idea* that ice reduces swelling. Obviously ice DOES NOT reduce swelling – it merely delays it – but, in any event, the key word here is "based."

But the fact that we all soon learned, courtesy of an article in the next day's New York Times, was that, "In this case, instead of using ice, doctors chilled Everett from the inside, infusing cold fluids into his veins. The treatment is experimental, though, and medical experts caution that it is impossible to say in an individual case whether it helped or hurt."

In sum, ice had nothing to do with it! NOTHING!

They even tricked me – until recently, I too had thought that they used ice!

But regardless, the ice gurus know that their days peddling the ice gospel are numbered, especially since the lay and university-based press have now started reporting the facts about their illusionary treatment option.

Indeed, because of this, they must see that the acceleration toward a post-ice world has entered overdrive – especially with the news-spreading efforts of some select bloggers.

Nonetheless, some seem to still be pretending that this isn't happening. Some others are probably busy writing new marketing material. And still others are most certainly hoping that this storm will just, somehow, pass.

But one thing is for sure: none of these people want to be a "guru" of a scientifically-rejected practice. They are most certainly longing for the opportunity to resume their roles as the *unquestionably* helpful "ice gurus."

Nevertheless, most of them will adapt – in time. But remember, there are still those who believe that bloodletting with leeches is based on a valid theory. Some even deny that germs exist!

It's time to add "Some even believe that ice reduces swelling" to that list.

Remember, people didn't always use ice on their injuries, and, in fact, its life cycle – while widespread and misguided – has been relatively short.

But we can all make amends with the facts now. After all, we are all supposed to get at least one mulligan, right?

I sure hope so, since I once voluntarily had a perm. A PERM!

The overwhelming vast majority of medicine has moved forward at light speed during the last few decades. Indeed, with today's medicine, the past is hardly a prologue, as rapid advancements that were not even imagined long ago have become commonplace.

But ice was always different.

It got to where it was by happenstance, not by merit.

It was sustained by lore, not facts.

And, most helpful of all to ice's rise is that it often got to operate outside of medical science. What a deal!

But that ride always had to end at some point.

And now it is about to.

Indeed, the shift to fact-based medicine became the ultimate enemy of ice.

News flash to the ice gurus ... the chill is gone!

Chapter 3

True Believers: Get In From the Cold

So, when it comes to issues of medicine and science, are you a "blind faith" true believer, or are you a "fact-based" true believer?

Do you believe whatever self-appointed "experts" say, or do you need proof before you believe?

If you were alive in the 1500s, do you think that you would have believed that the Earth was the center of the universe?

Or, are you more like Nicolaus Copernicus? Would you have joined him as he intently stared into the heavens and created complex mathematical formulas in search of the truth?

Knowing my personality, I suspect that I would have severely questioned the experts' notion once I had heard Copernicus' position.

But, unfortunately, that was not what most people living at this time did. Instead, the vast majority remained steadfastly committed to the "experts" view of the world.

Why? Well, the reason is really quite simple: virtually everyone else in the world accepted the "experts" ideas as the unequivocal truth. That blind faith belief had become ingrained in the collective human thought process as true, simply because that was "always" the dominating view.

Never mind that this view was not built upon scientific proof – it was just "accepted" because it for so long remained unchallenged. Worse yet, prior to Copernicus, any opponents of the experts' view were not able to provide anything more than their own, equally blind faith theory – a problem that opponents of ice shared up until the early 2000s.

Indeed, while I was not one of those exceedingly few opponents at the time, I can relate to their frustrations because even today, with the incontrovertible facts in my hand, I still occasionally face uphill battles.

Essentially, with no fact-based reason to cause people to believe otherwise, prevailing views – regardless of what their foundation was built upon – are exceedingly difficult to replace. And, as I have learned with icing, the fact is that even when opposing views possess the facts, it is STILL sometimes incredibly difficult to reverse *fake* "facts."

So, once there was fact-based reason to believe otherwise – thanks to Copernicus' effort to meticulously organize and present the facts – the previous blind faith belief seemed embarrassingly foolish.

Simply put, blind faith is no match for fact-based faith.

Indeed, there are many examples of the transition from blind faith to fact-based faith throughout medical history. Sometimes the transition is smoother than others and likewise, the period of change can range from swift to painfully slow – sometimes even negligently so.

Here are a few examples from the field of medicine that really put our icing transition in context.

Do you recognize the name, Dr. Ignaz Semmelweis? He is the one who figured out that doctors should wash their hands before surgery, especially if they just finished dissecting a rotting and/or diseased corpse.

It's creepy to even think that such a suggestion was ever even necessary – let alone controversial – but, at that point, it was actually spectacularly groundbreaking.

Semmelweis also introduced the idea of sterilizing surgery tools. Again, this sounds like a no-brainer, right?

Well, his suggestions were BITTERLY rejected by his fellow physicians.

Why? Well, his observations conflicted with the established scientific and medical "beliefs" of the time. As odd as it sounds by today's standards, the doctors simply did not believe that their filthy, contaminated hands and surgical tools could possibly be the cause someone to get sick.

Believe it or not, some doctors were actually offended by his suggestion – OFFENDED – that they should wash their hands.

This is a classic example of blind faith where people simply didn't know what they didn't know.

It was not until years later – when Louis Pasteur confirmed the germ theory and others finally began using the hygienic methods that Dr. Semmelweis recommended – that Semmelweis earned his rightful place in medical (and world) history.

Today, people have a clear understanding of the *actual* facts in this regard. And, as such, the importance of washing one's hands is thoroughly embraced not just by doctors, but by most everyone else as well. It took a while to evolve on this, but the fact-based faith has now roundly won the debate.

Here's another one. Do you know the original reason why barber shops had red and white swirly cylinders sitting on top of poles outside of their entrances?

The answer is stranger than fiction: to inform potential customers that their establishment offered bloodletting services.

Indeed, the red and white cylinder represented a bloody bandage and the pole represented the object that the customer would squeeze to effectuate greater bleeding.

But, as if this idea was not crazy enough in and of itself – why in the world would this responsibility lay with barbers?!

If people were going to do this, it seems like something that they might have wanted, oh, I don't know, a licensed doctor to perform this for them.

And relegated to the fringes it was not.

Indeed, it achieved wide popularity and its helpfulness was accepted as simple "fact."

It's a shame they didn't "know" to put ice on their (self-inflicted) wounds, then they could have been just perfect.

But, why barbers? Well, it made sense at the time. You know, on your big day out you could get yourself a snazzy haircut, and then, oh yeah, let a little blood!

It sure sounds crazy by today's standards, but bloodletting is actually one of the oldest medical techniques in history. It was once the most performed medical procedure in the world and dates back nearly 2,000 years.

So what did it treat? Well, like its freezing friend of today – almost ANYTHING!

Its application was utterly indiscriminate – asthma, indigestion, coma, diabetes, epilepsy, convulsions, gout, you name it; if you had something wrong, the "experts" "believed" that you just needed to let some blood. They were totally unaware of the (basic) physiological fact that blood moves all throughout the body, and thus, their very premise that cutting a "bad spot" would bleed only the "bad" blood from just that particular spot was totally wrong.

That sounds awful familiar, huh?

Twist your ankle, smash your head, break your arm, bump your knee, run to hard, lift too much, cycle too far – JUST ICE IT! It's the answer to *everything* injury or soreness related.

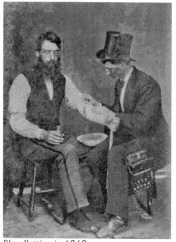
Bloodletting in 1860

For a moment, think about all of the injuries that you have either sustained or witnessed. Can you think of any instance in the last twenty years where ice was deemed inadvisable by any witnesses to the injury or would have been considered inappropriate by the purveyors of popular icing lore?

For many, such an instance is exceedingly hard to come up with, thanks in no small part to the collective "understanding" of icing.

Claims and corresponding societal "beliefs" of near-universal application should usually be sufficient cause for any skeptical (thinking) purchasers to *at least* question the general merits of the particular product – if for nothing else, just to ensure that they are not buying some bogus infomercial product.

Sure, duct tape, WD-40, aspirin, Vaseline, and various other products enjoy legitimate (and justifiable) wide-ranging uses, but such things are very rare in this world.

Anyway, back to bloodletting. So how exactly did it work, you wonder? Well, there were various ways to do it.

They – perhaps even your local barber – could cut you with a knife, poke you with a needle-like object, or attach a leach to your skin and allow the creature to suck your blood out.

Indeed, many of us have heard of the "leeches" technique, as it has secured its place in the public's memory of bizarre medical procedures of yesteryear.

But, how exactly did they determine when someone had "let" enough blood?

Well, when they passed out, of course!

The problem here is that the concept is based on entirely unjustifiable "science" and indeed a false premise. Bloodletting was based on the now-miserably discredited theory of the human body known as "Humorism."

Yeah, I know it sounds "funny" if only it weren't true. But interestingly, in some ways, icing damaged tissue is actually *even worse* than bloodletting. Why? Well because the inflammatory process's critical importance is a *well-known* scientific fact and, while bloodletting is *now* known to be insanely unjustified, no one at the time was aware of this.

And, as such, with this icing fact understood, the continued use of ice on damaged tissue is, actually, the equivalent of continuing to rely on an *already* fully discredited "fact." It would be like continuing to engage in bloodletting *after* humorism was rejected.

Like icing, no matter how bloodletting was done, no matter who performed the procedure, and no matter how advanced their equipment might have been, it didn't work. In fact, it often caused irreparable harm.

And, think again if you thought (hoped) that only the uneducated would consider participating in this bizarre process. Indeed, that was far from the case, as many members of the ruling class not only did it, but actually requested it!

Even President George Washington was a fan, and, sadly, not even his untouchable stature was sufficient to shield him from the *actual* facts of the procedure's merits.

Indeed, doctors now conclude that Washington likely died as a result of "over-letting." But, even if that was not the technical cause of his death, it certainly did not help that his doctors drained 3.75 liters of his blood in the ten-hour period just prior to his death!

Sounds like a bit much, even for supporters of letting, considering that the average adult male only has about five liters of blood in their entire body! That's 75% of his blood, gone in less than a day!

Not the severity, but the *extremity*, of this example actually reminds me of the icing supporters who encourage submersion in ice baths and full-body cryotherapy chambers. Oh well.

Anyway, the "experts" during this 2,000 year period truly *believed* that bloodletting was a legitimate medical treatment.

They *believed* that if they just provided the path, "bad" blood would just leak out.

Interestingly, their belief that bloodletting reduced blood pressure was actually sort of true. Indeed, if there is no blood, there is no pressure. But, of course, this also means that you die, which was not quite what they had in mind when they came up with this idea!

But, with bloodletting and ice alike, do not confuse "official" support with fact-based support. For example, bloodletting was still very popular until the end of the 1800s and was actually listed as a viable option in the 1923 edition of the textbook *The Principles and Practice of Medicine.*

The author of that book was Sir William Osler, the man considered to be the "Father of Modern Medicine." He was also the co-founder of Johns Hopkins Hospital. The point: don't confuse *official* with fact-based – they are not always harmonious.

Indeed, there are plenty of instances of blind faith medical procedures infiltrating "official" documents. And, unfortunately, ice is no exception.

Just look in nearly any physiology-related field's classroom. Ice is everywhere. It sure looks like an "officially" accepted method. The professors generally think it is. The students generally think it is.

And yet, despite this fact, soon the professors will not be teaching icing and the students will have no experience with it. Again: the facts about icing never changed – even if professors confidently taught it to their students on lots of expensive icing equipment.

Just like with bloodletting, the facts tripped up the "official" support for icing, and soon, both of these practices will be together in the same hazardous waste bucket.

Yet even more amazing with bloodletting is that, despite its millennium of prominence ending long ago and on an unceremoniously sour note, leeches are back!

But this time, their usage is extraordinarily narrow and is based on fact-based faith. Remember my story in the first chapter where Pat Croce had me freeze my foot so that I could stretch the tendon and heal?

While that was not necessarily "fact-based" – although it was based on well-established physiological principles – it was a legitimate and effective use of ice. It was an exceptionally narrow protocol and had nothing to do with the merits of icing damaged tissue.

Well, a similar case now exists with leeches. It turns out that leeches are an excellent way to drain blood from swollen faces, limbs and digits after reconstructive surgery.

I know, this is gross – and it is about to get grosser – but it is true!

Leeches are especially useful in keeping skin graft tissue healthy when reattaching small parts like ears. And here is a really cool piece of the puzzle: leech saliva is made up of more than thirty different proteins that, among other things, help to block pain and promote blood flow.

You see, despite their previous misusage, leeches are actually very clinically relevant. In fact, the FDA recently classified them as the first live medical device.

In sum, blind faith cannot intellectually compete with fact-based (evidence-based) faith.

Mere popular lore simply has no place in medicine – especially *after* there is adequate cause to believe the opposite through the lens of fact-based faith.

And, nearly everything that the "experts" have disseminated about the value of icing damaged tissue is the result of blind faith. Conversely, everything presented in this book regarding the "value" of icing damaged tissue is based solely on fact-based faith.

Think about it, how can you ever be sure that you make the best decision if you rely on blind faith? This is the case REGARDLESS as to whether there is fact-based evidence to the contrary.

Lacking proof to the contrary is a reality that we must all sometimes live with in our lives, but, fortunately, such is not the case with ice. Indeed, we are lucky to now have a plethora of evidence regarding the lacking merits of icing.

Finally, as I am sure that most others have as well, I have had numerous personal experiences relating to blind faith. While the following example has nothing to do with medicine, it is quite illustrative of the power – and, in this case, heartbreaking consequences – that blind faith can have. It serves as a stark reminder for me, and I hope that it will for you as well.

In July 1971 I was readying to enter my senior year of high

school.

I had set a goal to achieve something very important to me: breaking my school's long-standing pull-up record.

The rules were simple to follow; start from a dead hang (no swing, arms straight), bend your arms until your entire chin is high enough above the bar that you can see the tops of your hands, return to a dead hang, and repeat.

The number to beat was 41.

I had been secretly practicing since early spring, but now the time had come to put pressure on myself to stick with my plan. And there was only one way, of course, to ensure that my future self would not deviate from the plan: by announcing my goal to my buddies.

Since I knew that there was a pull-up bar around the back of the building, I decided to tell my friends in the place that we always hung out: in front of our school.

I proceeded to tell them that I could already do at least 25 pull-ups.

And, just as I predicted they would, one of the guys said, "Prove it."

So we went around back and I approached the pull-up bar.

I was ready.

I knew what I could do and I was ready to prove it.

The first twenty were simple.

The next five were tougher, but I still managed to complete them with relative ease.

Before I knew it, I had a new personal best: twenty-eight.

I felt great and truly believed that the record would be mine by the end of the year.

But, when school started in September, someone told one of my classmates, Frankie, about my goal and that they saw me do twenty-eight over the summer.

Frankie was built a lot like me but, considerably more muscular and a lot tougher.

In response to the news, Frankie announced that he too was planning on breaking the record, and that he could already do at least forty.

I was crushed.

I knew that there was no way to outdo him.

He was (obviously) way too far ahead for me to catch him.

As such, I abandoned my goal. I kept practicing, but completely lost focus of my record-breaking goal.

Several months later, we had tryouts for the Marine Physical Fitness Team – the national contest put on by the United States Marine Corp.

One of the events in the contest was – you guessed it – pull-ups.

Thirty (perfect) pull-ups earned a perfect score.

Both Frankie and I were trying out.

Coach Umberger said, "Reinl, you're up first."

I then approached the bar, jumped up, grabbed it, adjusted my grip, and began.

The first twenty were simple. But from there, it was tough – although not miserable.

I went on to complete thirty and achieve a perfect score.

The next couple guys didn't even break eighteen.

But Frankie was next.

I knew what to expect.

He would bang out thirty like it was nothing.

He approached the bar, jumped up, grabbed it, adjusted his grip and started.

To my complete and utter disbelief, Frankie was already struggling after just twelve pull-ups.

He ended up barely breaking 15.

I was sick to my stomach.

I had given up on my goal because I believed that Frankie was untouchable.

Blind faith had broken my dream.

From that moment forward, I tried my best to do all that I could to identify and reject any unsubstantiated claims – and became quite good at this.

I would go on to prove that pregnant women could, in fact, achieve greater comfort by building their strength and that mature senior seniors could, in fact, achieve greater mobility – indeed literally leave their walkers and wheel chairs behind – by building their strength.

Anyway, if only I had seen Frankie do pull-ups back in September, I would have known the truth and remained focused on my goal. Instead, I lost several months of needed practice.

It simply wasn't possible to focus on both the pull-up record and the intense daily training for the Marine Physical Fitness Team. I could only focus on one of them – and I was devoted to the team.

Not surprisingly, Frankie and I both made the team.

I ended up doing thirty pull ups in every meet and Frankie never got more than twenty.

In the semi-final round (the East Coast championships), I tied for first place overall. At the National meet, held at the Marine Corps base in Quantico, Virginia, I placed in the top twenty overall.

In case you are wondering, I still did end up trying to break that towering record of forty-one pull-ups.

I did thirty-nine.

After graduation, I suspect that Frankie never thought about that record again.

Conversely, I have thought about it thousands of times.

The lesson I now take from this: beware of blind faith.

Chapter 4

My Temperature's Rising!

So, were you ever an icing true believer?

Did you ever automatically think "ice" when you bumped your knee?

How about when you were watching a game on TV and a player sprained their ankle?

Or when a good friend told you that they had hurt their elbow playing tennis?

If yes, you are not alone.

The ice gurus of yesteryear did an amazing job convincing us all that ice was almost always the answer.

Somehow, they managed to get their message to the masses unchecked. But, in retrospect, while it was initially unlikely, such was the only viable path to wide acceptance of their protocols, since any "checking" of the facts would have invariably doomed their chances.

And, once they were successful, most of us saw little reason to believe otherwise.

But, in case you are wondering, I do not get to claim to have played the role of Nostradamus here either. I too got caught up in the ice storm. While hardly ever a fanatical ice-user, I did support icing for many years.

Indeed, in numerous instances, I used my (insanely cold) professional-grade ice pack on myself and encouraged my wife, daughter, son, and (now) daughter-in-law to use it on many other occasions.

I still clearly remember the first time that I used ice on something major with a family member. Before this instance, I had used ice on many comparatively smaller injuries, but never before on something so serious.

It was October 2003 and my wife had significantly injured her lower back at the gym. And, this was not one of those "it will okay in a few days" type of injury either. Indeed, it ended up taking several months before she was fully up and about.

Here's what happened. She had called me while I was away on a business trip and the tone of her voice instantly alerted me to the seriousness of the problem.

The nearly tear-inducing pain was so intense that she was literally forced to stop (nearly) all movement. Even simple trips to the bathroom became complicated endeavors requiring enormous effort and lots of assistance.

So, what did I advise her to do? Well, the first and most "obvious" thing that popped into my head was for her to have someone get our commercial-grade gel-filled cold pack – the kind that you would normally see in a therapy setting – out of the freezer.

Based on my general experience, this seemed to me the best option at the time. I then told her that I thought she would be best served by covering it with a thin towel and putting it on the tile floor.

I had figured that the hard floor would have been the best option to provide the needed support and keep the ice pack against her back.

I know that this sounds barbaric and cruel, but it was done with the best intentions. Further, it is not all that far removed from the *current* practices and beliefs of many physicians, therapists, and others.

Anyway, I was so focused on the tandem concerns of temporary pain relief and long-term healing, that I honestly hardly even considered the discomfort that she would have to endure between the freezing pack and cold, hard floor.

Fortunately (I suppose), she was in such pain that she was willing to do almost anything, and thus, the extreme discomfort did not deter her from my treatment suggestion.

So, I had her lay on her back with her knees bent, her feet flat on the floor, and the ice pack squarely covering her back for twenty minutes every hour until I was able to get home the next day.

However, I also encouraged her to try and gently move whatever she could as often as she could without ever causing additional pain.

I then proceeded to contact several of my orthopedic doctor buddies seeking additional advice before reaching what I thought was the best conclusion: that both the icing and the attempts to move the muscles needed to continue indefinitely.

When I returned home the next day, my wife was resting, albeit still not very comfortably. We continued the cold therapy for several days and immediately began adding various directed muscle activation exercises, such as having her press her back to the floor. With the same objective in mind, we also used our electrical muscle stimulation device.

As the days wore on, we continuously added more movements, as well as deep tissue massage. We were also still icing, but it was becoming much less of a focus.

And, let me tell you, this schedule remained intense even by my standards. Indeed, throughout the day, we worked on her back for about ten minutes on the hour, every hour. As you can imagine, this care was nearly around-the-clock and lasted for several weeks.

Ultimately, she fully recovered and actually ended up significantly stronger with more conditioned back muscles than she had prior to her injury.

As I was writing this section of the chapter, I talked with her about this decade-old experience.

Her memories are crystal clear.

And they are not fond.

Let me just preface my next comment by saying that my wife is well-aware of my current (general) position on icing.

Keeping in mind that both she and I fully acknowledge that what we did worked spectacularly well, you can see why it was very hard for me to answer her (highly-loaded) retrospective question, "If it happened again, would you still use the ice?"

In her mind, she was looking at this from two ways.

First, she was thinking that ice was part of the successful protocol and thus deduced that it may have helped in this process.

This is, of course, a mistake that many of us make all the time.

Just because we were ultimately successful with something *does not* mean that everything that we did to get to that result was helpful. Indeed, correlation does not always equal causation.

She did, of course, realize that there is simply no way – based on all of the incontrovertible facts about icing that she has been made aware of – that icing helped the healing process, but it was a tough question for me to swat away nonetheless.

So, we then carefully reviewed the facts about the healing process – as well as the procedures that we now know are best to do – and applied them to this particular circumstance. Quickly, the answer became obvious and unequivocal – ice was not a good plan.

Knowing that this would likely be the conclusion that we (I) were going reach, this answer led to the question that she really wanted to ask: "Why is the world then, did you have me lay on that freezing cold ice pack on the freezing cold tile floor!?"

Suffice it to say that I cringe at the very thought that I had her use an (already) provably unhelpful treatment "option," and can sympathize with her anger about the extreme suffering that came along with that process!

Anyway, with all that said, there is little doubt that the "ice" provided considerable temporary pain relief, especially during the first 24 hours when I was away.

Further, using the ice also provided a significant "psychological" advantage, since *believing* that we were addressing the problem surely made us both *feel* better.

But, as you would likely agree, none of those reasons comes anywhere close to justifying the intentional stifling of the healing process.

Common sense should have dictated that our main focus of activating the muscles (through movement and e-stim) was badly hindered every time that we used ice to do what ice always does: constrict the very vessels that the waste is trying to move through and slow the healing process!

For the next few years, I would go on to use ice on a number of smaller injuries without ever really questioning the merits of doing so. However, by 2013 – the next time that another major injury struck our household (this time, my fractured collarbone) – I was well aware about the perils of icing.

It was January 6th in Baltimore, MD, and I was out for a Sunday morning run when I tripped, fell, and broke my collarbone (e.g. it was not "cracked," but cleanly broken mid-shaft).

At this point, I was about a mile and a half from my hotel room. Another runner had seen my fall, but, by the time that she got over to help me, I had already figured out how to roll over and get back upright without using my hands.

When she arrived, she figured that I was seriously injured (I assume that the fall looked pretty bad based on her reaction) and readied to dial 9-1-1. However, before she could do so, I told her that my collarbone was indeed broken, but that I was otherwise fine and thus did not require emergency assistance.

Clearly a bit shocked at my answer, she then asked how I knew that it was broken, to which I replied, "Because I heard (and felt) the bone break."

She then asked what I was going to do and I told her that I was just going to run back to my (relatively) nearby hotel.

Upon hearing this (perplexing) answer, she insisted that I not run alone and asked if she could run back with me. I agreed.

But then, barely a hundred steps into our trek back to my hotel, I heard (and again, felt) another "crack."

The difference was, this time, it actually felt good. I just figured that it was the bone resetting.

Anyway, we then proceeded to run all the way back to the hotel. Once there, I thanked her for her help and we parted.

But, then, once I was inside of my hotel room, the comedy began. I really wish that I had this on video – I assure you that you would have found watching my tribulations thoroughly entertaining.

So, what made it so amusing? Well, have you ever tried to take off a tight-fitting sweatshirt with a broken collarbone without any assistance? If not, let me just say that it is a formidable challenge.

Indeed, I eventually found myself literally stuck with the sweatshirt three-quarters of the way over my head and my "compromised" arm lost somewhere in between.

At that point, I was deliberating between taking the elevator down to the lobby to ask for help and trying to call the concierge to see if someone was available to come to my room.

Fortunately for the sake of my dignity, I decided that neither option was appropriate and then proceeded to wrestle the sweatshirt off by myself.

Sure, I was determined in this regard, but, in retrospect this was actually an exceedingly bad idea. Nonetheless, it did prove to be a successful effort.

And, since I was in Baltimore and my favorite doctor was in the Philadelphia area, I decided to get my things together the best that I could and drive to him. I knew that I would be most comfortable having him be the one to do whatever action was necessary (including surgery) and so off I drove.

I was mentally prepared to drive, but that ended up not being my biggest challenge – for example, have you ever tried to pay a toll with a recently broken *left* collarbone?

Anyway, when I finally got to my hotel, the woman at the front desk asked me if I was okay. She had clearly sensed that something was wrong and I replied that I had broken my collarbone earlier in the day and just needed to get to my room.

She then asked if it hurt. My answer was something along the lines of, "Only when I move, but otherwise, it is not bad at all."

As you can probably imagine, that night was very uncomfortable, since lying down was simply out of the question and I had not yet learned how to sleep sitting propped up against the wall.

The next day, I called my doctor's office and he saw me at 1:00 p.m. Once there, he took an x-ray and confirmed that I had a mid-shaft break.

We then talked about what the appropriate next steps were and agreed on a plan. Following this, we proceeded to discuss the aftermath of the injury.

When he heard my "post-break" running story, he could do little else but look at me and ask, "Why did you run back to your hotel?"

A bit perplexed by his question, I replied with a look of serious confusion on my face, "What were my options?"

"You could've walked!" he replied

"Honestly, that option never crossed my mind," I then said.

Fortunately, I have known him for many decades and so he was not caught completely off-guard by exercise diehardedness.

Anyway, the next day, he arranged for me to see his partner (a shoulder specialist), who ultimately concluded that no surgery was needed.

This episode marked my first major personal test regarding icing since the avalanche of (new) information had so decidedly changed my views.

So, did I ever consider icing? Not a chance.

This served to confirm that, for the first time on a personal level, my brain was exclusively focused on evidence-based practices and no longer interested in the blind-faith "comfort" offered by any discredited – even if formerly ingrained – traditions of my past.

At this point, unlike during my wife's injury, I fully understood that the body's innate intelligence is *far* better at regulating the healing process than "I" am.

Does that mean that I did not take any action at all? NO!

Keeping in line with the body's healing process, I used my muscle activation device all throughout my healing process, beginning *immediately* after my sweatshirt debacle in my Baltimore hotel room.

This way, I was working to activate my muscles to help move along the waste (swelling) as quickly as possible without ever interfering with my body's healing process.

Indeed, this method is actually much easier and far more comfortable than constant voluntary activation (e.g. simply moving my arm around) in a situation like this when the goal is to help facilitate the movement of the "fluid" (swelling) that will otherwise accumulate in and around the damaged area.

Further, as I will explain in detail in chapter five, the amount of fluid sent to the damaged area is *not* an arbitrary or chaotic event and it is not there by mistake.

Instead, it is *precisely* the amount needed. And, the reason that it begins to accumulate is because of inadequate drainage – which is contingent upon muscle activation around the related lymphatic vessels – not because of any dysfunction in the healing process.

Anyway, I used my muscle activation device for more than sixteen of the first of thirty hours post-injury and five hours per day, every day, for the following three weeks. After that, I used it only on an as needed basis.

I also started functional movements within the first 48 hours, beginning with the involved fingers and hand before progressing along all the way to my arm and shoulder. But, keep in mind that most of these movements – especially in the very beginning – were exceedingly minor.

This was, however, perfectly okay, since that was all that I could do at the time. My only goal was to move whatever I could in as many non-pain-inducing directions as were feasible. I repeated this protocol literally dozens of times every day for the first month, gradually increasing the intensity and duration of the movements.

So, what was the result? Well, other than a slight, soon-to-pass, catch near the top of my reach (e.g. when I straightened my arms above my head), I had full range-of-motion by the sixth day post-injury. By the twenty-first day, I had resumed my normal distance running schedule and was back lifting weights the next day.

Keep in mind, that my healing schedule for this injury would be considered extremely rapid in nearly all circumstances. Most people would have iced the injury, which would have delayed the healing process, and would not have introduced movement anywhere near as soon, and, once they did, they would not have been as aggressive in carrying out their movement protocol (*because* of the painful swelling – which I did not have!).

Unfortunately, some degree of this vastly inferior icing/stillness protocol is what most people undertake. They are told to ice and by the time that they move, it is far too late to ensure optimal healing.

That reality is one of the things that I am truly hoping to change with this book, because such a protocol is a travesty. Remember, my body does not have some magical healing properties – indeed it is sixty years and tens-of-thousands of running miles old!

But, how did my treatment protocol work out in the long run? Well, I regained all of my strength within just a couple months, and, almost exactly five months post-injury, I ran my first marathon in more than thirty years – the day after my sixtieth birthday!

Not that it needs restating, but if I were given the opportunity to do it all over again, the answer to whether I would use ice is a resounding "NO!"

So, what happened in the intervening nine years that made me change my mind so decisively? Well, around 2006 I had decided that I wanted to work with the best of the best in professional sports.

I knew that I had a good message with regards to injury prevention and recovery, but I had no specific plan for exactly how I was going to break into the professional athletic scene.

Nonetheless, I was both determined and confident that I could figure it out. Sure, I was far from a complete outsider – as I had spent decades in the general business and had previous experience training professional and world-class athletes in my gym – but, I was well-aware that working full-time with professional athletes was an entirely different ballgame.

Indeed, I had been told by more than a few "insiders" that it was virtually impossible to get into professional locker rooms and even harder to stay there. And, that it was simply a matter of time, since there are only so many minutes in so many available days and everyone that sells this general type of product wants to get the "elites" on their customer list.

For example, during MLB spring training, there are only about fifty total days available to see the trainers and, before you even start, you can scratch about half of those days off of the list for various reasons, such as travel, team meetings, and player physicals.

Then, for the other twenty-five days, about two hours are set aside each day for trainers to meet with people like me (e.g. the hundreds of product and service vendors who want "in").

And, keep in mind that these trainers are very, very busy people and you must adapt to their schedules if you want a piece of the approximately fifty hours of vendor face time that each of them have available each year.

Here's a fun (but not that unusual) story to illustrate the point. I once met with the athletic training staff of the New York Yankees at 6:00 p.m. on a Sunday night in Tampa, Florida and then met with the athletic training staff of the Milwaukee Brewers in Phoenix, Arizona on Monday morning at 9:00 a.m.

Thus, after finishing with Yankees around 9:00 p.m., I grabbed something to eat before heading back to my hotel and then got up at 2:00 a.m. to catch a 5:00 a.m. flight to Phoenix, which arrived at around 8:00 a.m. (local time).

Why would I do this? Well, because that's what worked for them. All that you can do is take what you can get and do your best to make it work.

And, you can forget about the rest of the year, as it is virtually impossible to see trainers during the season – remember, they play 161 games in 182 days and about half of the games are away – and offseason availability is not much better.

So, here's what I did in the early years. I went to about two dozen trade shows and met with anyone who would meet with me in an effort to find out what exactly the head trainers, doctors, and athletes were buying and what they were actually using and why.

To this day, I still attend six to ten trade shows per year and personally meet with hundreds of team-affiliated trainers, doctors, and therapists, and carry on a seemingly never-ending email/phone conversation with at least 150 of them.

Here's what I quickly realized: the product buying list is really rather short and the "using" list is even shorter. Trying to explain and justify the reasons for why which products made the "buying" or "using" lists can be difficult (and indeed confusing), but, that is just the way that it is.

So, here's the reality: there are only a total of 122 head trainers in the NFL, MLB, NBA, and NHL *combined* and there are only about one-hundred other truly "elite" trainers. As a result of this exceedingly small universe, they almost all know (or know someone who knows) everyone else in the group. And, since there are only a few things that work best, good *and* bad news spreads very fast.

Further, due to the volatile nature of modern player retention, players moving from team to team help to spread any "news" even faster. Indeed, on several occasions, I have been called to meet with head trainers, who were, at the time, out of my "network," as the direct result of requests made by recently traded players who had been familiar with me.

Anyway, I just want to give you a quick feel of the above "small universe" story so you can understand exactly where I was coming from when I started.

Several years ago, I was asked by the head trainer of the Miami Heat (Jay Sabol) to meet with the head trainer of the University of Miami's men's basketball team (Wes Brown). When I arrived, I ended up also meeting with the head trainer of their football team (Vinny Scavo).

During the course of our conversation, Vinny asked me where I was going next and I told him that I was meeting with the head trainer of the Detroit Tigers.

He then immediately said, "Say hello to Kevin [Rand] for me. We used to work together at the Marlins, great guy, good friend."

Since that time, Kevin has personally recommended me to several other MLB head trainers and invited me back to spring training every year. In fact, this past year he even arranged for me to meet with his organization's entire minor league team of trainers.

Further, when I was there with those minor league trainers, one of them had seen a popular video about icing that I had done with Dr. Kelly Starrett (which I will explain in chapter six) and enthusiastically referenced that point during our meeting. My point: it is a small universe indeed.

Anyway, for the first five years, I kept a very low profile and rarely expressed my personal opinion absent a specific request from a trainer, and even then I was highly guarded.

During this time, I asked a lot of questions – especially with regards to products that the trainers said that they had used but did not like and products that they said they currently use and do like – and carefully listened to their answers, frequently taking lots of notes.

But, don't just think that I was a wallflower either. Indeed, I intently – some might say aggressively – interviewed many hundreds of these involved experts and read hundreds of related journal articles.

I also spoke at length to every product vendor who was willing to share their company story with me and read every word of every related marketing document that they offered me, including their company websites. Further, if it was possible for me to try their product, I tried it – often more than once.

Essentially, the purpose of this was to know all about everything that the pros were using (or considering using) so that I had a wide-range of personal experiences and knowledge about those products from which to draw whenever such information might be necessary.

This is where it gets really interesting.

My "try it" rule was simple: if they claimed that their product could reduce or eliminate pain and/or swelling, I wanted to try it.

As a result, I've been zapped by several different kinds of electromagnetic force fields, stimulated by at least a dozen different types of electrical stimulations devices – including one that caused such a violent series of contractions that my leg muscles literally hurt for a week and another that felt like thousands of bees were simultaneous stinging me over and over … ouch!

I have had ultrasonic sound waves shot through various parts of my body and used at least a half-dozen different strength lasers – including one that was so powerful that the caregiver and I each had to wear special goggles to protect our eyes.

I have had my legs compressed by what felt like two giant blood pressure cuffs and had various body parts pounded by handheld electrical thumping devices – including one (which cost over $2,000) that was so strong that I literally had to brace myself against the wall to remain in place, but which actually felt pretty good.

I have been frozen by a dozen or so different cryotherapy (ice) devices – including one that blew ice-cold air and only required a couple minutes of use each time – sat in what looked like a miniature space ship that is designed to provide high altitude pressure while remaining in place, had acupuncture needles stuck in various parts of my arms and legs, and been shook so hard on a stand-up vibrating machine that I nearly peed myself.

I have been bound up like a mummy with several different types of therapeutic tape and squeezed into various compression garments – including one upper body shirt that was so tight that I actually got trapped in it and required the assistance of the guy trying to sell it to get me out of it.

Additionally, I have smeared at least a dozen different types of "magic" gels, creams, and lotions on my legs and arms. Some of them smelled horrible while others felt disgustingly greasy. However, it was the one that contained some kind of "hot sauce" – which the guy selling it claimed that no one else used – that grabbed my attention more than the others.

You see, I found out the hard way why no one else used this "hot sauce" when I inadvertently touched my eyes after rubbing it on my legs.

After I made this terrible mistake, my eyes were immediately in agonizing pain and remained so for more than an hour. It honestly felt like someone was poking little hot needles in my corneas. Indeed, my eyes ended up remaining red for several days afterward. Interestingly, I never saw that particular product again.

I have even had two different therapists aggressively run a medal device that looks a little bit like a large polished butter knife over my hamstring muscles, which is purportedly used to breaks adhesions.

If you are wondering, the reason that I had it done twice was because the first time hurt so bad that I figured that it must have been done wrong.

Well, unfortunately for me, it wasn't "wrong," but actually the reality of the device. The result, both times, was extreme bruising and considerable post-treatment pain. Amazingly, this device is actually very popular and utilized by thousands of therapists and doctors.

Of course, this is just the highlights of my broad samplings, but I think you get the point: I tried stuff.

Anyway, here's what I learned. First and foremost, never make an unsubstantiatable claim. This is very important to always remember. Saying things that you can't prove turns people off and dampens your creditability.

Second, even if you can prove something, do not push your claim to the maximum or brag. Overpromising only sets you up for failure. The best method is to just tell the basic truth.

Next, do not trash-talk the competition; elite trainers generally hate that. In fact, I honestly believe that much of my success is attributable to the fact that I strictly follow this rule.

That said, I am more than willing to answer any questions and provide related evidence anytime the need arises. Indeed, the line might seem fine, but there is a very big difference between trash talk and telling the truth.

Lastly, if the head trainer of a professional athletic team or other elite trainer believes that your product could help them get their athlete "back in the game," they might talk to you. And then, if your way *sounds* better than what they are currently doing and is *believable*, they might give you a try.

Further, if your way *is* better, you're in – maybe. I say "maybe" simply because "better" does not always win. Indeed, sometimes tradition, familiarity, and/or ease of use trumps "better." And, if you are wondering, price is usually a nonfactor.

So why does any of this matter to you? Well, I want you to know that I wasn't just sitting in some ivory tower somewhere far away from the action before suddenly deciding to attack the ice gurus. In reality, that could not be further from the truth.

All told, I have flown more than two million miles domestically and spent nearly 1,800 nights – which amounts to about five total years – in hotels. Indeed, I am in the trenches and have been there for forty years.

And, what's more, I did not *ever* plan to discover that ice was an illusionary treatment option.

In fact, when I began this journey into professional athletics, I too used ice and believed that it was a legitimate treatment option (as I described earlier in this chapter).

And, in what is a bit ironic in retrospect, the first person that I asked for advice on how to become successful in world of elite athletics was, in fact, a bona fide ice guru.

Indeed, he represented the essence of success in this business, and, based on my own personal observations, seems to have sold more "ice" treatments to elite athletes than everyone else *combined*.

So, why did I pick him at that time? That's simple. I felt that since everyone who I wanted to meet and work with used – or at least owned – his ice product, learning his secret to success was imperative for me. At that time, he literally worked with every single team in the NFL, MLB, NBA, and NHL, along with numerous high-profile colleges and universities.

Keep in mind that this was in 2006, a time when I could easily fit my entire elite/professional trainer contact list on the back of my business card. Thus, he was, in my judgment, the best person for me to emulate.

Fortunately for me, he was willing to do all that he could to help me "break in" to the world of elite and professional athletics. Indeed, he very graciously, professionally, and painstakingly explained the market to me and provided excellent advice on what I should do.

He is an unselfishly great guy and, to this day, I thank him every time that I see him. But, ironically, his advice is what led me to ultimately crusade against icing and write this book.

So, what did he say to do? Well, he told me to never give up, tell the truth, and (I'm paraphrasing) to learn everything I could about how to eliminate pain and swelling and then sell that message.

But, why exclusively pain and swelling? Well, because it is the biggest problem! And, despite the fact that hundreds of vendors claim to have the solution, no one (fully) does and only a select few actually provide meaningful results.

Thus, since virtually everyone owned/used his product – which rather ingeniously combines the concepts of ice and compression – I read everything that I could find about how his product "eliminated pain and swelling" and asked every trainer that I spoke with to give me related feedback.

What I found was that his product's research articles were very well written and the results seemed equally impressive. And, most trainers openly acknowledged what the research proved: that his product was better than ice alone. Indeed, so far, so good.

But then, in a sincere effort to figure out what I could do to enhance the results produced by his product's dynamic duo (ice and compression), I read everything that I could find on the topics of pain and swelling and talked to several sports-medicine physicians and about a dozen professional team massage therapists regarding lymphatic drainage – the only viable way to eliminate swelling.

While many of these people were notable, my conversation with one such expert was particularly fruitful. His name was Mark Greenwood and his background was rather unique. He was a physical therapist and exercise physiologist, as well as a nationally-licensed massage therapist. His words were clear and unequivocal and served to crystalize and confirm what I had been hearing from so many others about lymphatic drainage.

This, in combination with everything else that I had learned, ultimately led me to a clear understanding of how the body eliminated swelling (which I will explain in detail in chapter five). And, most importantly, allowed me to understand precisely how eliminating swelling often significantly reduced/eliminated the cause of the pain.

This understanding of the proper action to take with regards to reducing swelling did, of course, stand in stark contrast to the results produced by icing – which amounted to little more than temporarily masking pain and often causing swelling to *increase.*

At this point, it became obvious to me that compression was the reason that his product got better results than ice alone. However, it also became obvious to me that compression alone would get even better results without any icing at all.

Further, I also recognized that the type of "passive" compression provided by this device was only *slightly* better than doing nothing at all. Here's why: ice slows everything down, (essentially) prevents lymphatic drainage, and can actually cause *more* swelling.

And, passive compression – meaning that there is no related muscle activation or subsequent signaling – which are needed to produce the natural flow of "supplies" and waste – is not only a sub-optimal method for moving swelling, it's not even a good method for doing so.

However, it was not as though I was onto some kind of breakthrough in the basic understandings of the physiological process. Indeed, that is far from the case, as the facts regarding lymphatic drainage are very well-know and clearly explained in countless textbooks and journal articles.

If you want further proof, you can do a little test. Take your right hand and grab your left wrist and squeeze it as hard as you can for one minute. Then, while you are still squeezing, ask yourself if the "compression" is improving circulation in and out of your left hand.

Thus, as you can probably imagine, this was a very uncomfortable time in my career. I had to decide if I was going to go along with the status quo that I knew to be wrong, or if I was going to point out the facts for the benefit of everyone that I talked to.

This decision was, however, not all that complicated, as I knew that I needed to do the right thing. So, I decided that I would recommend that both ice and compression should be avoided before, as well as during, any muscle activation techniques designed to eliminate swelling.

I did, however, still provide the following (soft) post-treatment recommendation, "Then, once you finish activating the athlete's muscles, use ice and compression if you feel that it is needed."

Then, as the years went by and fewer and fewer trainers were asking about ice and compression, I amended my recommendation to the following, "Then, once you finish activating the athlete's muscles, you likely won't feel that you need to use ice or compression."

Now, don't get me wrong: nearly every one of these trainers still, to this day, uses the ice/compression product. Most teams actually have several units, while a few have upwards of a half a dozen of them.

But, what really seems odd to me is that virtually everyone agrees that you should not use ice beyond the first 24-72 hours (depending upon who you talk to) if you are going to use it at all, and yet, many athletes use this product for weeks on end.

Somehow, many customers of this (expensive) product have become convinced that, since this product gets better results than ice alone, they should use it outside the ice gurus' own recommended guidelines.

I chalk all of this up to a gradual evolution. I realize that old habits die hard, but the fact that anyone still uses products such as this is hard for me to understand. Fortunately, with the use of both icing generally and this product specifically down considerably from just a few years ago, the ultimate outcome for these methods is really quite clear.

Chapter 5

Freeze Frame: Are Inflammation & Swelling Friends or Foes?

Let me first preface this chapter by saying that inflammation and swelling are NOT the same thing, they are not at all interchangeable, and they are not twins. If anything, swelling would be the (sort of) *evil* twin of inflammation.

Inflammation is your FRIEND and a critical part of the body's natural healing process, while "swelling" is your foe.

Of course, the increased fluid resulting from the inflammatory process that so often accumulates and "swells" is initially both natural and necessary, but when insufficient muscle activation allows the resulting waste to accumulate, it becomes problematic.

This process is not unlike the full bag of fresh groceries turning into a pile of trash – everyone wants the delicious food (the fluid), but no one wants it to remain for too long and become rotting garbage (the "swelling").

And, icing does nothing more than delay the inflammatory process while often allowing for *more* "swelling" to accumulate.

The problem, however, is that many have come to view "inflammation" as a dirty word, as an affliction that must be stopped at all costs. Well, such is the not at all the case, and this flawed premise has led to mass confusion about what inflammation actually is.

So what exactly is its purpose? I will be spending this chapter explaining the many of the essential aspects of inflammation and translating the complex process into lay terms.

First, let's begin with a hypothetical real-life scenario that we can use to understand the process from a perspective with which we are all quite familiar.

An NFL wide receiver is standing at the line of scrimmage.

He is mentally and physically preparing for the upcoming play.

The quarterback calls out an audible.

The play just changed.

The receiver is no longer a decoy and is now the likely target.

Wholly focused, he looks downfield.

As he assesses his opponents' formation, he is slightly distracted by an odd-shaped divot about six feet directly in front of him and makes a mental note to ensure that he avoids it.

The roar of the crowd is deafening.

The quarterback then flashes him a last-second hand signal as he regains his focus.

Seemingly without conscious effort, the receiver processes all of these minuscule details, knowing full-well that any of them could be the deciding factor in the success of the play, just as with any given play.

The center then hikes the ball to the quarterback and the play goes "live."

A linebacker quickly picks up on the play and points to alert the rest of the defense.

Upon catching the ball, the receiver is immediately hit hard by the linebacker.

He is nearly knocked to the ground.

For a split second, he mentally complains to the ref, *where's the flag?!*

Just then, he manages to regain his balance and focus.

Having broken the tackle, less than one second later he is running full speed down the field.

To avoid a speedy cornerback, he suddenly cuts right and then left before switching back right again.

His swift movement successfully juked the cornerback.

The total elapsed time since the snap of the ball is a mere 3.5 seconds.

The receiver has now run thirty yards downfield.

He then slightly turns to avoid three fast-approaching defensive players.

He then tightly secures the ball with his right hand and outstretches his left hand to fend off the threatening tacklers.

Less than a second later, he leaps into the air to try to muster a few extra yards.

As he soars through the air, defenders simultaneously hit him from the left and the right.

He promptly lands back on the ground.

Amazingly, he is being stabilized in the upright position thanks to the roughly proportional (crushing) force distributed relatively evenly to each side of his body.

Somehow he manages to remain standing after the defenders both fall to the ground.

The end zone is now in sight.

Determined as ever, he then tries to continue running.

But then, suddenly, for no immediately apparent reason, he collapses in agonizing pain.

His hand instantaneously wraps around his body as he grabs the back of his thigh.

Like so many athletes before him, he has torn something.

In his case, it is one of his hamstring muscles.

Now, just for a few moments, forget about this athlete.

Have you ever considered how many individual physical and mental actions are involved in this singular play for just this one player?

For those of us who have never played professional football, even the basic details are mindboggling. Just the act of processing all of the necessary visual and auditory information and then converting those directives into action is enough to fry the brains of many of us armchair quarterbacks.

Seriously, can you imagine trying to mentally process each

individual task, one by one, in the allotted time? There is a reason that there are just a few of them and millions of us!

And yet, this amazing feat is *nothing* compared to all of the interrelated neuromuscular and physiological processes needed to physically accomplish this act. Indeed, it is far too much for most of us to even try to decipher.

But wait, even as amazingly complex as those processes were during the initial running and maneuvering, even they are *simple* when compared to what is going on in the player's body as he lies on the ground trying his best not to move his leg.

You see, when his muscle tore, blood vessels ruptured and the inflammatory process instantaneously responded.

The escaping blood was immediately viewed as an emergency by his body.

Signals were sent to constrict the damaged vessels to limit blood loss. Other nearby vessels dilated (opened) to increase the flow of needed supplies to the area.

Simultaneously, his body was also building a clot, from the inside of the vessel out, to both stop leakage and hold the two ends of the damaged tissue together while the vessel was repaired.

Think about that for a minute. Using only what is readily available in the blood, the body builds a clot and begins to repair the damage. Amazing!

And, by the way, this clot is built lightning fast – usually within a couple of minutes – is spectacularly strong, and will self-destruct once the vessel is fully repaired.

Additional signals also summon specialized cells to the area to destroy germs and other foreign bodies. Other cells will also arrive shortly and then literally begin to ingest the related debris and prepare it for evacuation via the lymphatic drainage system.

This entire process is orchestrated and regulated astonishingly well. Indeed, it is literally in full-swing before the player even leaves the field.

But, for various reasons, almost everyone believes that they need to prevent, or at least limit, the inflammatory response related to tissue damage.

The problem is that the very premise of this belief ignores the universally-accepted medical fact that "inflammation" is phase one of the body's three-phase response to injury – a routinely *lifesaving* process!

Indeed, normal healing is *impossible* without the successful completion of *all three* phases.

This false belief also neglects the fact that the inflammatory process is a complex series of biochemically-driven processes that are naturally and automatically regulated by the body's innate intelligence.

And, these processes operate with such precision, focus, and speed that no computer or scientific research team in the world has yet been able to even begin to replicate them.

These processes also commence with amazing reaction time, initiating the moment that the damage occurs and ending the moment that the damage is fully mended. Oh, and the body operates this protocol without ANY outside influence!

For a moment, think about how incredible this is. The body launches this spectacularly complex reaction without any delays, second guessing, meetings, or voting – it just automatically and instantaneously turns itself on and off as needed.

The body INHERENTLY understands that the very first drop of blood resulting from the damaged tissue is sufficient cause to ring the alarm bells *long* before this rupture has the opportunity to cause enormous damage (e.g. ANY such internal damage could, ultimately, cause a person to "bleed out" if efforts are not made to clot a rupture).

So why does it do this? It is called self-preservation. If the damaged tissue simply went unchecked, you would likely develop a serious infection, if not die. Accordingly, any delay in the response is essentially considered by the body's innate intelligence to be an unacceptable risk.

The moment that damage occurs, the body responds by releasing a number of chemicals, such as histamine, prostaglandin, and kinins, at the very beginning of the inflammatory response.

Collectively, these chemicals cause an *increase* in (blood) circulation – via (now-dilated) nearby undamaged vessels – to the damaged area, which is necessary to bring in the "clean-up" and "repair" supplies.

They also act as critically important messengers that attract many of the body's natural defense cells (e.g. the "emergency response team" is sent to kill any invading germs and literally consume the problematic debris resulting from the injury).

This mechanism is known as chemotaxis – a process, by the way, that is obviously, *inherently,* hindered by the vessel constriction that necessarily results from icing!

Simultaneously, the body is *decreasing* – either by limiting or stopping – the flow of blood by *constricting* the *damaged* blood vessel(s).

This is done to achieve two important *sequential* objectives with regards to the constricted vessels.

The first is to temporarily slow, if not stop, the flow. The purpose of this part of the process – which is known as hemostasis – is to limit the related blood loss.

The second objective is to build a clot that stops the internal bleeding. The clot is (usually) completed in just a few minutes, a fact, by the way, which renders one of the core arguments of icing – that it helps to stop bleeding – essentially moot a mere 180 seconds after the injury!

Then, immediately upon the completion of the clot, blood flow resumes while the vessel(s) is/are under repair. Finally, once the repair(s) is/are finished, the clot(s) dissolve(s) through a self-destruction process.

Pretty impressive, huh?

And yet, we are supposed to believe that slapping something cold on our skin is helping this process?

If you are still not convinced, here is an amazing point regarding how the body actually manages to build the clot inside of the vessel and begins the general repair outside of the vessel.

The clot is created by a stunning series of events that are so complex that it seems almost impossible that the human body can even manage it from the inside – let alone through external action with an ice pack from the top of the skin!

This series of events *automatically* comingles von Willebrand's Factor, platelets, adenosine diphosphate (ADP), platelet thromboplastin (Factor III), fibrin, red blood cells, and a host of other "ingredients" to prevent continued internal bleeding.

Immediately after this series of events, what I call the "emergency response" and "clean-up" teams start to arrive in the general area.

Yes, these leukocytes have technical names, such as macrophages and neutrophils, but my simple names very accurately describe the missions of these varying subdivisions of the body's life-saving white blood cells.

The "emergency response" team (neutrophils) is the first to arrive at the site of the injury. Their job is to neutralize harmful bacteria and (possibly) signal satellite cells.

The "clean-up" team (macrophages) then arrives and aides the healing process by surrounding bacteria and dead cells before ingesting them to clear the area for new cells to grow.

Within days, phase two of the healing process is (well) under way as fibroblasts (collagen producing cells) begin to construct a new collagen matrix, which acts as the framework for new tissue cells.

Once most of the debris is removed, the damaged area begins to develop new blood-carrying capillaries through a process known as angiogenesis or revascularization (which, by the way, is enhanced by muscle activation, not by stillness).

Once blood flow to the damaged area is adequately reestablished, the repair of the damaged tissue – or phase two of the healing process – is well underway.

Remember, all of this occurs *automatically* – (fortunately) meaning that there is NO need – or even justification – for interference.

Finally, phase three of the healing process – which is known as remodeling – begins.

While this phase can literally take months or even years to complete, the *external* effort to help repair the tissue should commence as quickly as possible.

Indeed, the introduction of gradually increasing levels of stress is an imperative action to take. Preferably, you should do whatever movements that you can, no matter how slight, that *do not* induce pain (assuming that your doctor agrees).

And, keep in mind, that failure to do this will necessarily prevent optimal healing, likely cause dysfunctional scaring, and negatively impact future function.

While there are certainly more known details about the three-phase process than I described above, I must say that I nonetheless view this entire process as an utterly inexplicable living miracle that always needs to be thoroughly remembered when dealing with an injury.

I say this because there are simply too many unknowns for me, or anyone else for that matter, to be able to *fully* explain the healing process. However, if you are interested in learning more about these processes, you can easily find additional information in many medical textbooks as well as various (recently) published peer-reviewed journal articles.

That said, my above explanation is a good place to start and sufficiently detailed for this discussion. After all, no matter how much information is used to understand this conclusion, the bottom line is that inflammation is a *good* thing and we *need* it to survive.

This fact is indisputable, but, over the years, I have found far, far too many people who are formally trained (and highly competent) in this general field who "know" this information, but fail to adequately *remember* it. Thus, for some of you, just adequately "remembering" stuff that you already "know" will be all that you need!

Once these basic facts about inflammation are understood, the entire discussion about what to do post-injury, especially with regards to icing, is easy to recognize. But, like I said before, too many people – experts and lay persons alike – either do not know about this aspect of the healing process or do not apply it when determining how to handle injury.

Indeed, once this process is universally understood, very, very few will actually believe that they are more "qualified" to regulate phase one (the inflammatory phase) of this complex process than their body's innate intelligence – with nothing more than a small block of ice no less! Sometimes facts really are odder than fiction.

But, what do medical experts on the topic of inflammation say? Do they believe that it is okay to significantly delay, modify, or (try to) skip the inflammatory phase of the healing process? What are the incontrovertible facts related to this topic?

Well, although there are a wide variety of sources that explain the same general answers to these questions, below I have referenced two of the most concise, well-referenced explanations that I am aware of, each of which is consistent with related clinical textbooks and other published evidenced-based material.

The first is from a September/October 1999 article in the Journal of American Academy of Orthopedic Surgeons entitled, *"Loading of healing bone, fibrous tissue, and muscle: implications for orthopedic practice."* It goes as follows:

> *"Healing, the tissue response that can restore tissue structure and function after injury, results from a complex, interrelated series of cellular, humoral, and vascular events.*
>
> *"Tissue damage and hemorrhage caused by injury or surgery initiate a response that includes inflammation (the*

cellular and vascular response to injury), repair (the replacement of necrotic or damaged tissue by new cells and matrix), and remodeling (the reshaping and reorganizing of repair tissue).

"This continuous sequence of events begins with the release of inflammatory mediators and ends when remodeling of the repair tissue reaches a homeostatic state."

The second is from a January 2003 article in The Physician and Sportsmedicine entitled, *"NSAIDs and Musculoskeletal Treatment What Is the Clinical Evidence?"* It goes as follows:

"A major rationale for using NSAIDs in the treatment of musculoskeletal injuries has been their anti-inflammatory quality. The prevailing argument is that healthy tissue is not inflamed; therefore, if we stop the inflammation in an injured tissue, the tissue will be healthy.

"The problem with this viewpoint is that, in addition to being a sign of injury, inflammation is a necessary component of the healing process. As noted by Leadbetter **'inflammation can occur without healing, but healing cannot occur without inflammation.'**

"Whether the injured tissue is a ligament, tendon, or muscle, the body responds to injury with a sequence of events that begins with an influx of inflammatory cells and blood. The inflammatory cells remove debris and recruit cytokines and other growth factors toward the injury site.

"This inflammatory phase is partly mediated by the same prostaglandins that are blocked by NSAIDs. In a healthy healing process, a proliferative [repair] phase consisting of a mixture of inflammatory cells and fibroblasts naturally follows the inflammatory phase.

"The fibroblasts build a new extracellular matrix and persist into the final phase of repair, the maturation [remodel] phase, where, if all goes well, functional tissue is laid down. The key point is that each phase of repair is necessary for the subsequent phase."

Finally, let me leave you with a quote regarding the process of the lymphatic system from the *Textbook of Medical Physiology's* explanation: *"The lymphatic system is a 'scavenger' system that removes excess fluid, protein molecules, debris, and other matter from the tissue spaces. When fluid enters the terminal lymphatic capillaries, any motion in the tissues that intermittently compresses the lymphatic capillaries propels the lymph forward through the lymphatic system, eventually emptying the lymph back into the circulation."*

Okay, now for the question that I nearly *always* get: what about SWELLING?

Many people mistakenly believe that "swelling" *is* inflammation. It is not. Swelling is simply the accumulation of fluid in a given area (e.g. the site of an injury).

This mistaken thought that "swelling" is inflammation has caused widespread confusion. Indeed, this belief has negatively impacted the careers of many aspiring and accomplished athletes alike.

How you ask? Well, it led many people to *attempt* to *prevent* inflammation – thinking that it was swelling (the problem) – which only served to delay, or worse, prevent optimal healing.

Oddly, however, the most prevalent technique in this regard – icing the damaged tissue – neither prevents inflammation nor helps to reduce swelling.

In fact, icing only temporarily *delays* inflammation and much of the time actually causes *more* swelling, not less. Accordingly, it does precisely *nothing* to contribute to the evacuation of "swelling."

This basic medical fact has been so glazed over for so long that many people now seem to have a hard time accepting it as the truth. Indeed, once the ice is removed from damaged tissue and normal body temperature at the site of the injury is restored, the inflammatory response resumes (thank goodness!).

But seriously, what are people thinking? Do they just figure that the body somehow "forgets" what it was doing before someone interrupted this lifesaving process by using ice to freeze (and therefore constrict) the passageways that it uses to get supplies to the injury site, especially when this is the ONLY method by which the body can keep itself alive?

This might lead you to believe that there is *nothing* good about swelling. Well, it is true that this all seems to paint a rather negative picture of swelling, but that is not *exactly* the case. Think of it this way: you want fluid to get there – because that means that the inflammatory response is doing its job – but you also want it to leave as quickly as possible.

Increased fluid is, after all, a necessary and fundamental component of phase one of the healing process. And, contrary to popular belief, the amount of fluid sent to the damaged area is not an arbitrary or chaotic event.

Instead, it is a vigilantly regulated process designed to help the body regain a homeostatic state, a process that ultimately depends on the lymphatic system to move the fluid and other waste away from the damaged area and back into general circulation.

It is true that trapped "waste" sometimes triggers the inflammatory response, which then sends more fluid to the damaged area. But, generally speaking, this is NOT because there is too much swelling, but rather because there is too little lymphatic drainage. And, this issue is (obviously) best settled by doing a better job evacuating the waste, not by stifling the healing process.

That last point is very important to understand. Swelling is simply the *accumulation* of waste at the *end* of the inflammatory cycle. And, this accumulation is due entirely to the lymphatic system's failure to evacuate the waste – a process that can *only* be accelerated through muscle activation.

Indeed, if you optimally move the fluid, excess amounts do not accumulate, period. Indeed, believing that swelling is the problem is akin to blaming the water that is trapped in your bathtub because you failed to open the drain. If you just open your tub's drainage system, the water will go away.

Likewise, if you open, or "activate," your lymphatic system, "swelling" will go away. And, similarly in both cases, the wider and longer that you open the drain, the faster the drainage will occur.

But you still might be wondering if icing helps to move waste. The answer is a resounding "no," and here's why: ice *slows* everything down. It abates, or worse, shuts off the signals between the nerves and the muscles, which effectively forces the cessation of lymphatic drainage – the only means by which the body has to reduce swelling.

Indeed, the lymphatic system works best when the surrounding muscles contract and relax, and thus, when there is no muscle action, there is little or no drainage. Remember, the lymphatic system is basically a *passive* system.

And, worse yet, whenever ice is used, it can actually *increase* waste in the area because it causes the lymphatic vessels to backflow.

The following is an excellent explanation of the well-known medical fact from a 1986 article from the journal Sports Medicine entitled, *"The use of cryotherapy in sports injuries."*

> *"When ice is applied to a body part for a prolonged period, nearby lymphatic vessels begin to dramatically increase their permeability (lymphatic vessels are 'dead-end' tubes which ordinarily help carry excess tissue fluids back into the cardiovascular system).*
>
> *"As lymphatic permeability is enhanced, large amounts of fluid begin to pour from the lymphatics 'in the wrong direction' (into the injured area), increasing the amount of local swelling and pressure and potentially contributing to greater pain."*

Furthermore, icing can easily cause additional damage. Besides the commonly known issues related to frostbite, icing can also cause general tissue damage. This fact was well-documented in 2013 National Strength and Conditioning Association article entitled, *"Topical cooling (icing) delays recovery from eccentric exercise-induced muscle damage."*

The authors of the peer-reviewed and indexed study said, *"These data suggest that topical cooling, a commonly used clinical intervention appears to not improve but rather delay recovery from eccentric exercise-induced muscle damage."*

So then, what is the best way to prevent swelling? Well, there are two ways that work very well: blocking it from the front end or evacuating it out of the back end.

The former occurs with the use of anti-inflammatory drugs. The basic idea of this inherently unnatural method is to prevent the inflammatory response altogether. Obviously, this is (usually) a very bad idea.

The latter, however, is the body's natural method, which facilitates healing (e.g. lymphatic drainage).

Remember the explanation of the lymphatic system from the *Textbook of Medical Physiology, "The lymphatic system is a 'scavenger' system that removes excess fluid, protein molecules, debris, and other matter from the tissue spaces. When fluid enters the terminal lymphatic capillaries, any motion in the tissues that intermittently compresses the lymphatic capillaries propels the lymph forward through the lymphatic system, eventually emptying the lymph back into the circulation."*

When considering all of these facts, the old idiom of "walk it off" is still, in principal, a very good idea. But, of course, I am not suggesting that you (always) *literally* walk it off. Instead, I am merely noting the need to *activate* the muscles around the damaged tissue in any way that you *safely* can.

In fact, I'll even add in my new adapted idiom: "Use your brain, never cause pain."

So, here are the two things that we know for sure regarding what you should do post-injury: (1) if you do nothing, the damaged tissue will swell, hurt, atrophy, undesirably scar, and heal slowly; and (2) icing, at best, grants nothing more than (potential) minor, temporary pain relief, and, at worst, it actually causes additional damage.

Thus, if your ankle is swollen and your doctor has recommended controlled movement, you should try to slightly wiggle your big toe. Once that feels good, try to add part or all of your foot and/or lower leg.

Once you can do that, try to partially weight-bear. Then, try to take a few steps using a cane or other like-device. After safely achieving that, go for a short walk ... and so on.

Just always remember that your goal is to activate as many of the muscles around the damaged tissue as possible without causing any increased pain or damage.

Indeed, this is the *only* way to evacuate the otherwise trapped waste (swelling) and thus, the faster that you are able to safely activate the largest number of nearby muscles, the faster that the swelling will go away. It is simple "lymphatics."

I know I am, but are you hooked on "lymphatics?" Once you are, optimal healing is sure to ensue!

So then, why then do so many people, even today, believe that icing reduces swelling? Well, as I began to explain in chapter one, you can trace the origins of this illusionary treatment option back to the first reattachment of a severed body part.

The media, for more than twenty years, pushed the "put ice on severed body parts to preserve the detached tissue" story to the public, who, regardless of the facts, eventually believed that they "heard" that they were supposed to put ice on all damaged tissue.

And, somewhere in the beginning of that twenty year period, many people started putting ice on the still-attached portion of the severed body part.

For example, wherever index fingers were detached, people learned to put both the severed body part AND the involved hand on ice as soon as they got the bleeding under control by elevating, remaining still, resting, and/or using compression techniques, such as tourniquets or hand pressure.

And, this protocol for severed body parts – which has now become ingrained in the public psyche – is incredibly smart. Since ice delays the body's natural inflammatory response to damage, it correspondingly (temporarily) significantly limits swelling. And, in this case, that is a *very* good thing, since swelling can badly complicate the reattachment process.

The side-effect of this understanding, however, has become very problematic. People generally now think that inflammation and swelling are the same thing and that both are equally bad for *all* injuries.

Indeed, this practice of putting ice on the intact body part is likely what started the misguided "belief" that putting ice on, for example, a pulled hamstring, would stop the internal bleeding and therefore help with the injury.

But, this overlooks one little explosive fact: the body's innate intelligence stops the bleeding *automatically* within a few minutes via the inflammatory process, which I explained in detail earlier in this chapter.

Nonetheless, through this lens, it is easy to see why so many people believe that ice is the reason why their injury stopped bleeding internally.

Furthermore, the "severed body part protocol" – compression, elevation, rest, and ice – led directly to the (once) popular protocol explained in the acronym "RICE" – which stands for rest, ice, compression, and elevation.

Indeed, the RICE protocol makes a lot of sense if you cut off your finger, but no sense for a sprain on the very same finger. Truly, the misapplication of RICE is epically disastrous.

In summary, icing *does* help preserve detached tissue and limit swelling, etc. in the still-attached portion of the body part, and thus remains a brilliant idea when dealing with a severed body part.

But, with that said, the reason that ice is such a great idea in this setting is because the detached body part is no longer attached to the body and will therefore rapidly rot and die if external action is not taken.

And, likewise, limiting swelling, etc. – even though it is done by delaying the inflammatory process – at the site of the injury is a very good idea because of how much it easier that it makes reattachment.

Indeed, the reason that icing is such a great idea in this regard (e.g. the suspension of the healing process) is precisely the reason why it should never be used on any other athletic injury.

But, unfortunately, far too many people have merged these two polar opposite issues and thereby advocated the wrong protocol for the vast majority of athletic injuries.

Indeed, the reasons for icing a detached body part have precisely nothing to do with putting ice on a torn hamstring muscle, or a sprained ankle.

Chapter 6

The End of the "Ice Age"

For me, the end of the "ice age" officially came on August 7, 2012. That was the day that Dr. Kelly Starrett (of CrossFit fame) posted the video of his interview with me on his popular "MobilityWod" blog.

We had recorded the low-budget video a few weeks prior at the 2012 CrossFit Games (the world championships of CrossFit) in Los Angeles, CA, the Games' annual home.

In the interview, Dr. Starrett had me explain to his audience – whom he affectionately refers to as "leopards" – why I say that ice is an illusionary treatment option.

The interview was inspired by, and indeed based on, an article/report that I co-authored and posted on my website (www.GaryReinl.com) in June of 2012 entitled *"Anti" Inflammatory*.

The article had made its way around numerous professional athletic trainers, but, up until that point, its impact was relatively modest and confined to my network of elites.

I had met Dr. Starrett earlier in the year at his famously basic CrossFit Training Center in San Francisco, California. It was then and there that I provided a detailed explanation about the broader objectives of icing and gave a related hands-on demonstration that Dr. Starrett not only understood and embraced, but actually used as the basis for changing the way that he practiced medicine from literally that point forward.

It is noteworthy to mention, however, that it was actually very easy to convince Dr. Starrett icing damaged tissue was nearly always a bad idea. Indeed, he had begun questioning its value long before we met and started scaling back his use of ice years ago. Additionally, he had always been aligned with the hands-on muscle activation portion of my presentation.

So, what did I tell and show him? Well, since the detailed contents of our interaction are comprehensively covered in chapter five, I will just provide a condensed explanation of the very basics of the interplay between ice, inflammation, and swelling. The fundamentals of our conversation went as follows:

I asked, "Why do people use ice?"

The response, "Inflammation."

I asked, "To get more of it, less of it, or keep it the same?"

The response, "Less, of course."

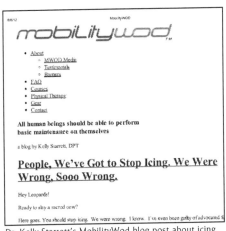

Dr. Kelly Starrett's MobilityWod blog post about icing

I asked, "Why would anyone want less inflammation? Don't they agree that inflammation is phase one of the universally recognized three-phase healing process (e.g. inflammation, repair, remodel) and that without it, optimal healing is impossible?"

The response, "Well of course, but they don't want all of that swelling."

I asked, "So they do want the inflammation, they just don't want the swelling?"

The response, "Correct."

I asked, "Okay, since swelling is essentially the accumulation of waste at the end of the inflammatory cycle, the only way to move that waste is via the lymphatic system, and the lymphatic system is basically a passive system nearly fully reliant on muscle activation around the lymphatic vessels; how could shutting off the signals between the muscles and the nerves, which is precisely what happens when you ice damaged tissue, accomplish that task?"

The response, "It doesn't."

Debate over.

And away we went!

Within a few days, the word was out and I had drawn first blood.

Never again could I only tell part of the story. Never again could I customize my presentation to fit within any particular customer's comfort zone. Indeed, within weeks the video had been viewed more than fifty-thousand times.

Shortly thereafter, that number climbed to more than ninety-thousand. However, suddenly, a noticeable split amongst the "leopards" began to form.

Two distinct viewer reactions became glaringly apparent, and most everyone seemed to fall pretty firmly into one of the two camps: those in agreement and those in disagreement.

At first, the ratio of supporters to skeptics was about 20-1 (in my favor). But, as the news spread and numerous well-known bloggers joined our side of the debate, the skeptics simply "melted" away.

For most of the relatively few who had been presented with this information, but were still trying to begrudgingly hold onto the now discredited "facts" about icing, the proof simply proved too overwhelming.

They certainly saw the mass epiphany happening all around them, but I assume that this was just too much, too soon for them to handle. They were simply unable to accept that such obvious facts ruled the day against the world's most prevalent injury treatment option.

After all, how could conventional wisdom possibly prove so miserably wrong – and indeed utterly inept at recognizing basic facts – about something so fundamental?

The benefits of icing couldn't be a myth! After all, Earth is both flat and the center of the universe, right? Remember, those beliefs lasted much longer than icing will and believers were much more fervent about their positions on a much more foundational aspect of human existence!

But, as this message began to really take hold, opposing positions began to go "cold." That is not to say that people did not rigorously question my rationale – believe me they did! Honest questions still remained, but they were always (easily) answerable and did not ever dominate my conversations.

Indeed, by late August 2012, I was spending at least ten hours each week on the phone with doctors, trainers, therapists, and athletes who called me as a result of the video.

One such call came from Scott Caulfield, the head strength coach/performance center manager at the National Strength and Conditioning Association's headquarters in Colorado Springs, Colorado.

Scott told me how he really enjoyed the video and also pointed out that his organization's journal had published an article online just that month detailing how ice delays recovery. He even remarked how amazing it was that so many people did not know this information.

Anyway, some of these people called to simply thank me for opening their eyes about the merits of ice. However, many others called to

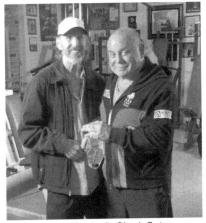

With John Schaeffer, Apolo Ohno's Trainer

express their appreciation for confirming what they had privately suspected based on their years of personal experience.

These people now felt that they possessed both solid evidence and a coherent explanation of the previously disparate (even if plentiful) evidence to share with their ice-supporting (addicted) athletes, clients, patients, friends, teammates, and colleagues.

It was as though this was the video that so many were waiting for to liberate their own private beliefs and, at last, allow them to bring their friends "in from the cold."

Thanks to Dr. Starrett's undeniable credibility and my simple organization of the related facts, people finally had "permission" to tell the truth about the icing of damaged tissue.

Indeed, it was truly a modern day version of *The Emperor's New Clothes* – Hans Christian Andersen's classic 1887 Danish fairytale wherein everyone pretends that ice is both useful and helpful.

Like the child in the story, once I pronounced that, "Ice is an illusionary treatment option," everyone became willing to admit the truth and felt empowered to speak up and join me.

However, whereas the only harm in the earlier version was a naked emperor, in this modern version, the harm is serious, widespread, and frequent. That is the naked truth about topical icing.

Anyway, by mid-September 2012, things really started to heat up – in more ways than one. While attending the outdoor demonstration part of cycling's seminal annual event known as Interbike, "it" happened.

The event is held in Bootleg Canyon, a world famous cycling park just west of the Hoover Dam in the rugged Mohave Desert. The scorching temperatures – which consistently hovered around 100 degrees as I fought to withstand the heat in the all-day outdoor event – were just as unforgiving as the surrounding terrain.

There was as much dust as there were cyclists, and I was standing alone somewhere between the hot dog stand and the registration tent. I was thirsty, sweating, and uncomfortable – and so was most everyone else. But not even these conditions could shield the video from finding me.

Indeed, without warning or any invitation, a young man approached me with his hand extended.

As I reached out to greet him, he said to me, "You're Gary Reinl, the guy from Kelly's video, I recognize you. Your interview was awesome! Who knew? Cool, really cool, thank you."

And that was just the beginning.

By the end of the five-day event, another dozen or so well-wishers thanked me for the video.

"It" had happened.

The word was out.

My simple message was no longer confined to elite training rooms.

The boundary had been broken. Now regular athletes were hearing this critical information that had previously been reserved exclusively for professional and world-class athletes.

And, strangely enough, my simple organization of these glaringly obvious facts turned me into a bit of a revolutionary (and perhaps heretic for the last few remaining stragglers).

Despite the fact that this information has been there, right under everyone's noses for many years, thanks to a simple presentation, I was now recognizable outside the world of elite athletics. Indeed, I was now the face of the opposition to the world's most prevalent injury response method.

By the beginning of December, nearly everyone that I spoke with was aware of my argument about icing – whether they saw my video with

Dr. Starrett, read my *"Anti" Inflammatory* paper, had been informed of my position through conversation with their peers, or some combination thereof.

From this point forward, I almost always had to address this issue early in any conversation, which often led to long, detailed personalized explanations of the facts about icing.

In fact, around this time, at the Major League Baseball Trainers' meeting in Nashville, TN, this was a big topic of discussion. Indeed, at least one trainer (usually two or more) from practically every single MLB team had positive things to say about my "anti-icing" position and made it a focal point of our conversation.

After my presentation to the trainers, the words of one assistant trainer from the Chicago Cubs summed up the sentiment in the room very well.

He said, "This really makes sense. I get it. This really makes sense."

By the end of the MLB meeting, I had been invited to visit twenty-six of the thirty MLB teams during spring training. It was then that I realized that my decision to use my interview with Dr. Starrett to introduce this issue to the public was a good one.

However, taking this from theory to practice in the training room required immense fortitude from the trainers entrusted with treating injured players.

One such example occurred with Ken Crenshaw, the head trainer of the Arizona Diamondbacks, a man whom I had already been working with for several years by that point.

Ken told me how he sold the idea of going "iceless" to his pitchers who had long since made the use of ice part of their second nature. Keep in mind that nearly every MLB pitcher has been told since they were in little league to put ice on their shoulder following any throwing session.

Indeed, this icy response to sore shoulders was so ingrained in the culture that it had become the instinctive response, the oh-so-obvious – and rarely, if ever, ever questioned – default action.

Consequently, nearly every time one of Ken's pitchers finished a throwing session, they asked him for some ice. So then, how did Ken break this harmful cycle and bring the pitchers in from the "cold?"

Well, after putting them on a muscle activation device for thirty to forty-five minutes, he would tell them to go get a hot shower, and then add that, once they were finished, they could stop by on their way out to get iced.

The first couple of times, the pitchers did indeed stop by for their icing fix, but then, as Ken proudly told me, they simply stopped asking.

This was a great example of this truly amazing transition. Guys who had gotten "iced" since they were little kids (subconsciously) changed their attitudes when they unwittingly experienced firsthand that the benefits of ice were completely illusionary.

Indeed, my introduction of this message was actually surprisingly short, thanks to an obviously hungry public who relentlessly thrust this issue forward at a breakneck pace.

When I recorded the video, I thought that it was time for the public to hear this information. But, as it turns out, this message was actually long overdue, as shown by the rapid embrace by so many grateful athletes and trainers.

I had spent much of my career trying to help athletes be their best, dating all the way back to the early 1970s when I trained many elite athletes in my gym, but this message was, by far, the biggest help that I have ever provided to athletes.

They had been grossly misinformed, their "go-to treatment option" was meritless, and I could help. As a lifelong runner who had spent many years using ice just like everyone else, I can say that this fact alone made this video not just a good idea, but a great idea.

There is one point here, however, that I must clarify. I had mentioned that nearly everyone whom I had spoken with had heard my message one way or another.

Well, it is important to understand that at least 95% of my time is spent working with trainers and physicians who provide care to professional and world-class athletes. Thus, my universe of clients, while comprised of very impressive and influential people, is actually quite small.

Remember, as I said before, there are but 122 head trainers between the NFL, MLB, NBA, and NHL – thirty-two in the NFL and thirty in each the MLB, NBA, and NHL. And then, if you add in all of the assistant trainers, team physicians and chiropractors, and all the other "elites" that I work with, my total number of clients is only about 500.

Thus, of the millions of ice-using athletes in the U.S., these trainers are barely responsible for a few thousand of them.

But, while this number is small, the group is also very tight and extremely interconnected. And, this group does a very good job at policing who gets "in." Essentially, if you are "in," you are really "in." And, conversely, if you are not "in," you are unlikely to see the inside of any pro training rooms.

My point is that information, especially when it is controversial and potentially ground-breaking, spreads fast amongst this group and, based on the response, can quickly determine if you get to stay "in."

Well, initially this group found my position on ice to be a bit unconventional. However, as time went on and this message sunk in, the exact opposite became true.

Sure, I had to take this debate into the lion's den of training rooms and provide many details to convince these very smart men to change their attitudes about ice, but their knowledge of the human body's physiological properties coupled with their general open-mindedness joined forces to knock ice off of its frozen pedestal.

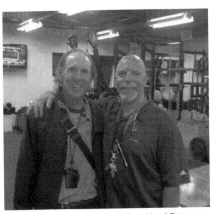

With Gary Vitti, Los Angeles Lakers Head Trainer

Indeed, in nearly all of my interactions with these trainers, once the details were hashed out, it was abundantly clear that the emperor was naked. Their full acknowledgement of the facts about ice then came in short order and, once that occurred, this message was no longer unconventional.

Amazingly, today if you tried to convince one of these elite trainers to put ice on a swollen ankle, you would likely find the trainer trying to help you understand the related facts about icing. But still, if you were to insist, they would likely just thank you, smile, and walk away.

By January 8, 2013, the circle that began with the posting of the video with Dr. Starrett began to close.

I was sitting in the Havertown, PA, office of Dr. Nicholas DiNubile of "DrNick.com" fame, who also happened to be my lead co-author on the *"Anti" Inflammatory* paper, along with my film crew.

We had just completed an hour-long interview with Dr. Nick on the topics of injury prevention and post-trauma recovery. Ironically, just one day prior I was an (unexpected) patient of Dr. Nick after I fell in Baltimore, MD, while running and broke my collarbone (I had been in town for the 26th Annual Baseball Medicine Conference).

And no, I did not request ice nor did Dr. Nick recommend it!

But anyway, it was then that Dr. Nick told me about the (in)famous call that he received regarding "Kelly's video."

Dr. Nick had been called by the clinical director for his group's eight therapy clinics to speak at a meeting with the group's entire therapy team.

However, they did not want their nationally-known sports medicine expert, best-selling author, and Chief Medical Officer of the American Council on Exercise to talk about his orthopedic expertise. Instead, much to Dr. Nick's befuddlement, they wanted him to talk about "Kelly's video."

The message had made its way out of professional locker rooms and all the way down to a local meeting between a doctor and his extended team. It just so happened that this doctor was also very close to the original paper that inspired the video! Not that Dr. Nick was unhappy about this, but I was absolutely ecstatic!

So, the next day I met with John Schaeffer – the world-famous trainer of such Olympians as Apolo Ohno and Louie Vito, as well as a plethora of other professional and world-class athletes.

John himself is also a world-champion heavyweight kickboxer and holder of numerous powerlifting world records. As such, his opinions are formed as both an elite athlete and trainer of elite athletes.

I had known John for several years, and he had long been well-aware of my position on icing, but I had never before asked him about his views on the topic.

When I asked him about his icing usage, he looked at me as only John can look at someone and said, "I don't have ice here, wouldn't use it if I did ... haven't used it in years. Doesn't work."

A few days later, as my trek around the country conducting interviews continued, I met with Tim Clark, the (then) head trainer of the NHL's Anaheim Ducks, whom I had been working with for years.

His comment to me served as a harbinger for what would soon become the general temperature around a league that's very existence revolves around "ice" (but I suppose that I do not object to gliding atop the frigid pest in a victory lap over my icy nemesis).

His simple words, "We don't use as much ice as we used to," reflected the barometric reading that I had been trying for months to achieve.

I had been working very hard to get hockey players "off the ice" and that was finally becoming a reality!

Anyway, by late January, spring training was unofficially underway and I was invited. I spent my weeks flying back and forth between Florida and Arizona in a near continuous loop.

By the end of March I had met with the head trainers, assistant trainers, and rehabilitation coordinators of nearly every MLB team, as well as about twenty-five minor league teams. By the time that April rolled around, my "anti-ice" message had caught fire.

Then, on April 11, 2013, I received a call from Roger Caplinger, the former head trainer of the Milwaukee Brewers and now medical director for the entire Brewers Baseball organization, which said it all.

His exact words before saying goodbye and ending our conversation were, "Each day we are using less and less ice."

Although Roger's closing comment seems like the ideal spot to end this chapter, I want to add a few quick stories from my spring training excursions.

While I deal almost entirely with professional athletics, I was invited to meet with trainers from three universities, and, since I was able to fit them into my chaotic schedule, I agreed to meet with them.

My first stop was Lynn University. The head trainer had called me after watching Kelly's video and, while I had never heard of the school before it played host to one of the 2012 Presidential debates a few months prior, it seemed like a good opportunity.

I had an early a.m. meeting that morning with the St. Louis Cardinals trainers at their nearby facility and was able to fit the Lynn trainers in before flying to the NFL trainers meeting in Indianapolis, which takes place each year the day before the NFL combine begins.

Upon my arrival, Lynn's head trainer assembled a half-dozen coaches and fellow trainers in their treatment room. This was quite a different scene than I had ever before experienced, as each member of the university staff had already seen (or at least heard about) my video with Dr. Starrett.

I had grown so accustomed to preaching my "anti-ice" gospel to skeptical audiences that it was honestly a bit odd for me not having to convince anyone of anything.

I was actually a bit nervous. After all, I had grown so comfortable taking my arguments to icing supporters that I almost did not know how to talk to those already supportive of my anti-ice message. However, as I quickly learned, the message spoke for itself and the meeting went great.

My second foray during this stretch into the university locker room came at Arizona State University. Much like at Lynn, the men's basketball head trainer had seen the video and cited it as his reason for calling me. He had arranged for the head trainer of the women's basketball team to join us, and the three of us had a great meeting.

Upon its conclusion, I immediately went to meet with the trainers for the Oakland A's minor league system. I already worked with the A's major league trainers, but I had never met with the minor league trainers.

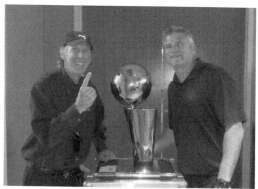

To my continued amazement, several of these trainers lavished me with even more praise about the video.

With my sole objective of helping athletes never relinquishing its position from the forefront of my brain, I could not help but

With Jay Sabol, Head Athletic Trainer of the Miami Heat

feel that this day had been a great one.

My final collegiate meeting, this time at the University of Miami, was vastly different from the previous two, primarily because I already had a long-standing relationship with several trainers at the school thanks to an introduction from Miami Heat head trainer, Jay Sabol.

Thus, the head trainers of the men's and women's basketball teams – as well as the head trainer of the football team – already knew my view of ice.

As such, in this instance, I was just stopping by to say hello and personally congratulate the head trainer of the men's basketball team on their recent Atlantic Coast Conference (ACC) championship. And, truth be told, I also wanted to get a glimpse of their new sports training room.

However, after a brief fifteen-minute meeting with the director, I was asked to speak to a couple of assistant trainers in the main treatment area. The next thing I knew, I was presenting to about a dozen University of Miami students.

This went so well that a few days later I received a call from one of the trainers who wanted to know if I would come and speak to all of the school's athletic training students. Happy to spread the word to the next generation, I humbly accepted.

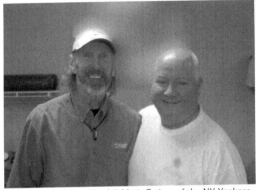
With Steve Donahue, Head Athletic Trainer of the NY Yankees

So now, not only was this message getting to students, it was also beginning to rapidly spread rapidly to other sports as well. That was about the best news that I could have ever hoped for.

Indeed, the day before my meeting at the University of Miami, I had spent several hours with David Donatucci, the Director of the Institute of Performance at the PGA National Resort & Spa.

While this was not my first meeting with David, I mention it because he really gets this message and he is helping accelerate its spread among the ranks of professional golfers.

It was, however, the three days following my meeting at the University of Miami that served as the gratifying capstone of my tiresome whirlwind of a journey around the country.

During this time I met with the trainers for the Detroit Tigers minor league team (I had previously only worked with their major league counterparts), the Houston Astros, and, finally, the New York Yankees.

I mention this because my experience with this trip to the Yankees was much cooler than ice could ever be.

During my locker room meeting with Yankees head trainer and good friend, Steve Donahue, everything stopped.

It was moments like this that drew me into sports as a young boy.

Of course, it was still about the athlete, but this time, it was much bigger than any flawed injury response method, no matter how widespread it might be.

It was Mariano Rivera, one of the greatest pitchers in baseball history, getting ready to call it a career. The press conference was just down the hall in the pavilion behind the third base stands right there at Steinbrenner Field.

The entire team – players, coaches, trainers, everyone – followed him down the hall. It was such an amazing sight to see up close that, for those few minutes at least, my months-long sleep deprivation did nothing to make me feel tired. It was sights like this that made me feel that my relentless crusade to help athletes was completely worthwhile.

A few hours later when Mr. Rivera walked on to the field to pitch, he received an extended, breathtaking, and well-deserved standing ovation. It was quite the scene for a legendary champion and I am grateful to have witnessed it firsthand.

And, also roughly around this time, another legendary champion, this time in the form of Gary Vitti, the Los Angeles Lakers head trainer, wanted to meet with me. I have known Gary for many years, and thus he knows my views on most everything related to injury response very well.

When I arrived, he gave me a detailed explanation of a treatment protocol for a muscle activation device that proved extremely successful for one of his star athletes.

When he was finished, I could not help but comment, "Ah, no ice. I like that."

To which Gary immediately replied, "I know, you don't like ice."

I loved it. Simply hearing the eight-time champion's voice mention my position without prompting was awesome.

My arguments had reached just about every trainer in the four major American sports and my position was well-known to just about all of them. It had become inescapable not because of me, but because the facts are so impossible to argue with.

Okay, it is now late April and the circle is about to close.

While, at a sports science symposium in Colorado Springs, CO, where I was meeting with Dr. Summers, the Director of Sports Medicine for the U.S. National Fencing Team and the Team Physician for the 2016 Olympics, he and a group of third-year students from his university listened to my presentation.

When I was finished, he not only made arrangements for me to provide my alternative to ice for his athletes, he had the Director of Sports Medicine from his university (the Southern California University of Health Sciences) come speak with me.

Shortly thereafter, the director invited me to meet with his entire staff at his university's sports medicine center. The message was now spreading back and forth and all around between professional athletics, collegiate athletics, and Olympic sports.

Okay, seriously, this is it ... the circle is almost entirely closed. But first, I need to quickly comment on my experience at this year's NFL trainer's meeting. However, since this was the eighth consecutive time that I had attended this annual meeting, most of the trainers already knew my position on ice, and thus this meeting was actually more of a social gathering for me.

Nonetheless, I retold my story to everyone who wanted to hear it and even found a couple of new guys that I had never spoken to before. No one – and I mean literally no one – even remotely suggested that my position on ice was the slightest bit wrong.

This was truly a great tribute to the effort that I put forth to inform NFL trainers about icing. I could not have been happier!

And, then finally, on April 25, 2013, I received a call from a barber in New York, who, completely unbeknownst to him, had his call (re)directed to me.

His sore muscles were not the result of athletic exertion, but rather of cutting hair, a task that can really take its toll after a while!

He said to me, "Hey you're the guy from the video ... I recognize your voice."

Circle closed.

But wait ... it eventually reopens and there are three more things that I just have to share with you!

First off, I was at the annual national meeting of the National Strength and Conditioning Association (NSCA) when a very energetic young man named Will Hooper stopped me and said, "You're the guy from the video. My professor, Dr. Nick Bacon (Ph.D., CSCS, HFS), at Belmont University Department of Sport Science used your video in my class as a teaching tool. It's a great video, thank you."

After an hour-long multi-dimensional conversation about the video (which ultimately involved at least a dozen other NSCA community members), Will asked if he could get his picture taken with me to show to his professor.

I, of course, agreed and requested that he ask his professor to contact me. Sure enough, when Dr. Bacon contacted me, he confirmed the story, and also added, "I would love an advance copy [of ICED!] if possible and perhaps to use your text in my S&C [Strength & Conditioning] courses."

Well, I must say, that is the exact response that I was hoping for!

Next, I was invited to speak at the American Chiropractic Association Sports Council's Annual Symposium. My topic was, you guessed it, recovery.

Since only one doctor openly disagreed with me during my talk and well over a hundred told me afterwards that what I had to say really made sense, I was very happy with my presentation.

Oh, and by the way, after privately speaking for over an hour with the guy who repeatedly interrupted my talk, I am happy to report that he seemed to have had an epiphany near the end of our discussion.

Anyway, another young man named Matthew DiLallo (M.A., CSCS, USAW) approached me and told me that his entry in the student poster presentation contest was based on my video with Kelly and proved that RICE was wrong.

I ultimately talked with him (and his friend) for about an hour, and, I must say, even though this kind of thing happens to me all the time, it never gets old. I simply love speaking and interacting with the next generation of leaders.

And here is my prediction: Mathew WILL make a difference and so will the many others just like him.

Finally, I was speaking with my neighbor, Jay Thompson (who is my age), just before "ICED!" went to press.

Up until that point, he knew nothing about my book (or position on icing) and so, when he asked what the book was about, I asked him, "Have you ever heard that you should ice your knee if you hurt it?"

Immediately, he replied, "Sure, but don't do it. It will slow everything down. It's not good."

When I asked him how he knew that, he said, "Well, I was national champion roller skate dancer back in the eighties and my coach [Bob Labriola], who had produced more champions than anyone else ever or since, always told us that ice was bad and to stay away from it.

"In fact, he had a saying that he always said to his athletes, 'Never do a cool down after dancing. Instead, do a *warm* down. Cool downs make you stiff now and hurt later.'"

Now that's cool!

Circle closed now (for now at least).

Chapter 7

The Cold Truth About Ice Gurus

"First they ignore you, then they laugh at you, then they fight you, then you win." –Mahatma Gandhi

While I remain skeptical of the suggestion, it is possible that the "ice gurus" are honest and sincere in their (continued) professed beliefs as to the legitimacy of their products and protocols.

And, while I find this exceedingly hard to believe, people in the icing profession may well be totally unaware of the basic physiological effects of their products. I would think that people in a field as narrow as icing would know next to everything about it, but maybe I simply expect too much.

Perhaps they remain (intentionally) ignorant and are totally unaware that making injured tissue cold unequivocally and indisputably delays the healing process, prevents or significantly delays lymphatic drainage, and often ultimately causes further damage.

They may just be responding to the market demand for such products, and, in the process, inadvertently preying on a wholly unsuspecting public.

I suppose that it's even possible that none of them know the truth, that none of them know that they are selling snake oil – which is defined as, "Something that is claimed to be a solution to a medical problem, but is not effective."

However, regardless of their culpability, and just like the snake oil salesmen of yesteryear that roamed the American Frontier, they push a method (icing), which is entirely unregulated by law or the medical profession, on an innocent public.

And, ironically, if ice *were* a regulated over-the-counter (OTC) medical product, it would likely never get cleared for use by the Food and Drug Administration (FDA).

Why? Well, to get cleared for such use, manufacturers need to prove, among other things, effectiveness and safety (e.g. that their products do not cause harm).

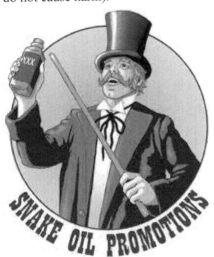

Ice would miserably fail the effectiveness test, as there are literally no peer-reviewed studies that prove any such effect. And, the contradictions, precautions, and warnings (e.g. frostbite, increased muscle damage, etc.), needed to comply with the "do no harm" portion of the clearance process would almost certainly push ice into obscurity as a prescription-only product.

But, fortunately for the ice gurus, the medical profession is not about to attempt to regulate the use of ice. Besides the fact that such a feat would be nearly impossible – as virtually everyone maintains direct, unrestricted access to ice – physicians are far too busy managing other medical issues to focus on frozen snake oil.

Anyway, as the story goes, the original "snake oil" was derived from a topical preparation made from the Chinese Water Snake and used by Chinese laborers to treat joint pain.

The preparation was promoted in North America by travelling salesmen, who often used accomplices in the audience to proclaim the benefits of the preparation.

Interestingly, however, most "snake oil" sold in the U.S. had nothing whatsoever to do with snakes. Alas, the original snake oil salesmen didn't even really sell snake oil!

At least the ice gurus use ice – or, at a minimum, something that feels cold. I guess, in an odd way, that makes them more credible than their forefathers, even if their product causes harm whereas the original snake oil was a mere sham.

Further, the ice gurus, like their predecessors, earn their money by persuading people to accept the benefits of their various products, which, at their core, represent false information. But, as I said, it is entirely possible that any particular "ice guru" has no idea that they are selling snake oil.

In fact, I too once believed that *ice was nice.*

No doubt, the pomp and circumstance that insulate this procedure from reality is seasoned and coarse. Nonetheless, and again, like their predecessors, they almost always require their customers to pay cash up front.

This might not look unseemly until you consider this next fact. You see, when insurance companies stopped paying for ice treatments in the 1990s – and rationally-thinking people simultaneously refused to self-pay for such treatment – most therapy clinics stopped the routine use of ice.

This cessation of mass icing was abrupt; despite the fact that it had been previously sold as essential treatment.

Surprise, surprise, ice was never really needed after all ... hmmm.

By the way, I personally mark this as the official beginning of the end of the "ice age."

But it gets worse.

While they generally stopped using ice at this time, it still remains a sliver of their treatment protocol. And when do they use it? Well, almost always post-treatment. That is not to say that its usage pre-treatment is a good idea, but let's think about the merits of using it post-treatment for a moment.

First, they "treat" you, which means that they do something to you or help your body do something for itself. This "something" likely causes some degree of micro-trauma, which is a positive thing, assuming that your caregiver is capable. This micro-trauma then sets into motion an inflammatory response designed to "clean up the mess" and repair the damage.

The success of this inflammatory process is, of course, contingent upon circulation, essentially "good stuff in, bad stuff out."

Thus, since ice inherently prevents normal circulation, you might want to question your caregiver if they try to affix a bag of ice to your newly-damaged tissue with twenty feet of Saran® wrap.

But in any event, these ice gurus are very well-funded and organized. And make no mistake, icing damaged tissue is big business.

How big, you wonder?

Well, it is hard to tell exactly, but, nearly every institution of higher learning that offers any kind of "medical training" (e.g. physical therapy, occupational therapy, athletic training, exercise science, recreational therapy, or sports medicine programs) has all or most of paraphernalia related to "icing" damaged tissue.

There are ice machines, ice packs, chemically-filled cold packs, vapocoolant sprays, cold tubs, whole body cryotherapy chambers, devices that run very cold water through sleeves that are custom made for knees, ankles, and shoulders, and there are even devices that blow very cold air.

And, since each institution needs to simultaneously prepare numerous students for the "real" world, they often possess multiple brands of each item.

I was tempted to not comment on the "whole body cryotherapy chamber," but since this is likely the best example of what can go wrong when you give the ice gurus money and let them "figure" stuff out, I just had to say something.

I suppose that it's reasonable to assume that, given the often inadequate (by their standards) performance record of ice cubes, the ice gurus figured that the problem with ice was that it is too small, to warm, and too cheap.

So what was their solution?

Something bigger, colder, and much more expensive, of course!

Before we get to the physiological merits, let's just start with a quick dose of common sense. With temperatures down around -166 degrees Fahrenheit, it can literally cause frostbite in mere minutes – a disheartening fact (unfortunately) proven through what they call "user error."

So far I am interested, how about you?

Well, unfortunately, for Manny Harris, he was interested in this tool and paid dearly for it. You see, in 2012 he suffered a freezer burn so bad that it actually cost him his spot on the Cleveland Cavaliers, who decided that the best course of action was to waive Harris and sign someone else.

A similar situation occurred with Olympic gold medal-winning sprinter Justin Gatlin, who was prevented from competing in the 2011 world championships as a result of the injuries that he sustained from the device.

Anyway, when you enter the chamber, they blow liquid nitrogen-cooled air all over your body. While I personally question the safety and wisdom of breathing ultra-freezing nitrogen-cooled air, it actually gets much worse than that.

After less than five minutes spent in the chamber, it is claimed that the user will then enjoy faster recovery. I will let you deduce your own conclusion on this one. Simply put: this is so silly that meaningful comment is not possible for me.

It does, however, remind me of a witticism that my mentor, Arthur Jones – the inventor and founder of Nautilus® – frequently told about the gurus who so often take society in the wrong direction.

His story is called, "One Less Bump."

Here's the point behind the title. Before the wheel was round, it was, of course, square. But the wheel gurus, who were very wise and all-knowing had determined that the problem was the four bumps that came with each revolution.

For most of us, that seems like a reasonable, even obvious diagnosis.

So then, what did they do? You guessed it, they made a triangularly shaped wheel ... *one less bump*!

The problem was that their "solution" went in the wrong direction! The right direction was MORE sides allowing for *smaller* bumps!

They should have progressed to pentagonal, hexagonal, heptagonal, and octagonal shaped wheels, which would have invariably led them to the ultimate solution: a circular wheel!

But no, they saw the problem with the original invention – just as everyone else did – and they "solved" one of the bumps!

Unfortunately, the ice gurus suffer from the same thought process. Heck, I'd even say that the whole body cryotherapy chamber knocked off another bump! Alas, just what we were waiting for: a two-sided wheel (is that even possible?).

From here, there's no way that it could get worse, right? Well, this next one might just represent the official devolution to no wheel at all. That is not because it is worse than ice – in fact it is not – but because it is mindlessly viewed as the solution – even the healing savior!

And how did it earn this distinction? That's simple. You see, even as it earns the same "F" as ice alone, it comes a bit closer to the apparently coveted "D-" than does ice alone.

Here's the deal: normal compression therapy rarely solves the problem, but, unlike ice, it does not ever really "set you back" either. And, on occasion it can actually be of miniscule assistance. Thus, when competing head-to-head with ice, it wins every time against its often harmful opponent.

One company – by far the most successful and biggest financial player in the therapeutic ice business – has a combination unit. It simultaneously makes your damaged tissue cold and compresses the area though a very sophisticated computer driven pneumatic pump.

They proudly claim that their device is the "first-ever sports medicine and post-op recovery device that simultaneously delivers active pneumatic compression and adjustable cold therapies."

This is so obviously unwise that I imagine that the reason no one else had previously done this was because it was such a flagrantly terrible idea.

My simple question is, how could the makers of this $5,000 ice/compression device not understand the fundamental principles of fluid dynamics? Do they actually believe, regarding the movement of waste (swelling), that compressing ice-cold tissue is better than compressing normal temperature tissue?

Seriously, think about this for two seconds. If I handed you two tubes of toothpaste – one at normal body temperature and one fresh out of the freezer – and then asked you squeeze out the toothpaste, which one would be easier to empty?

How about if you had two bottles of water – one frozen and one at room temperature – and asked you to turn them both upside down. Which one would drain faster?

Come on, you know they know. Or do they? Take a close look at their research and their related claims. Their primary goal is to simply outperform ice alone. And, in study after study, they do!

They have repeatedly proven that combining compression and ice is better than ice alone. Well great, that is just what we were waiting for – the coveted "D-" solution!

The big problem is that currently "everyone" uses their "superior" product. They have testimonials, videos, and celebrity endorsements. Essentially, ignorance is bliss.

But, since the very core of icing is now shown to be nothing more than an illusionary treatment option, I highly suspect that the makers of these products will soon be finding new lines of work and that their products will end up exclusively in museums, such as the Museum of Questionable Medical Devices.

And, while I am not sure how fast such exhibits will come into existence, I do know that the faster that the word gets around, the faster it will happen. It is as simple as that.

But, before that time, I suspect that the makers of these devices will suggest that my claims are preposterous, ridiculous, and that only they and their like-minded ice evangelizers are sufficiently qualified to comment on this "highly-sophisticated" topic. They will probably encourage you to ignore this book and throw it away.

That is what the gurus do every time that anyone puts forth a new, superior idea that they did not first think of. That is always how it works, but it can take time.

Fortunately, however, things move much faster in today's world then they did in the time when it was first suggested that Earth was not the center of the universe and the sun did not revolve around the Earth.

But now, let's get back to the students – the future leaders.

Not only do intuitions of higher learning buy vast assortments of icing "items," they must also create courses to teach the students how and when to use each item.

As such, this requires books, seminars, protocols, worksheets, labs, and, let's not forget, professors – the experts with the greatest potential for positive influence but also the greatest power over students whom they can fail for disagreeing with "facts."

All of this generates lots of tuition fees and opens the flood gates to the Holy Grail of academia – grant money – which is provided in large part by the ice gurus!

See the problem? The status quo remains in a constant state of reinforcement even as the objective facts remain diametrically opposed to the claims made by ice gurus. But, depending on one's viewpoint, there is one terrifying/encouraging situation here.

And, what might that be? Well, there are vast cracks in the collective scholastic thought on this topic. Even the academic status quo is badly confused – mostly because facts often get in the way of this wholly unjustified treatment method. And I am not talking about healthy disagreement. Rather, I am referring to outright intellectual and practical chaos.

What do I mean? Well, after forty years of widespread use, even the ice-supporting academics can't agree on much of anything other than the general lore that "ice helps."

With no consensus emerging, they have yet to coalesce on seemingly basic questions, such as what protocols should be, which types of injuries are appropriate for icing, how soon post-injury to administer ice, how long each icing session should last, how often a particular injury should be iced, what the depth of penetration should be, how to accommodate wildly varying levels of adipose tissue, and what to do about hugely differing degrees of depth in tissue damage – which alone begs the glaring question: how could applying ice over a deep bone bruise possibly help the related damage to the bone without causing damage to the superficial tissue, since it is a well-known fact that ice severely damages skin and all other superficial tissue when it becomes too cold?

And, none of this even speaks to the most fundamental question of all: *when* is icing no longer advisable? Theories in this regard range from mere minutes to several days. Oh boy.

This has developed a wild bunch of ideas, with some even claiming that the best option is a well-administered five-minute massage with a frozen cup of water with the top edge of a paper cup torn off, of course.

Anyway, more than a few are far ahead of me on this topic and stopped using ice years ago, even as I was using ice on myself, my wife, and my kids. But, unfortunately, many more have simply invested far too much effort to even consider the voluntary abandonment of ice and incredulously scoff at the simplicity suggested by the icing counterargument.

Think about this pragmatically; it is not easy to be incorrect on a foundational argument and it is even harder to admit as much. We are talking about invitations to speak at national conventions, opportunities to write articles and books, offers from reporters to give interviews, the ability to conduct seminars, the capacity to award continuing education credits, chances at departmental promotions, access grant money, and, really, entire careers.

Now, since the students spend so much time (and money) learning how to talk the talk and how to use all of this ice paraphernalia, and, while attending graduate school, were likely either directly or indirectly involved with related research, what do you think they do when they finally graduate from school, pass their state licensing exam, get a job in a clinic that owns many thousands of dollars of icing "stuff," and their clinical director wants everyone iced before they leave the treatment area?

That last question was a trick.

Let's try it again: what do you think that recent graduate will do when you say: "Why do you want to put ice on my damaged tissue? Do you honestly believe that my body's natural inflammatory process is a mistake? That you, with your little bag of ice and roll of Saran® wrap, are more qualified to regulate this universally recognized lifesaving process than my body's innate intelligence?

"Do you understand the principles of fluid dynamics and the subsequent movement of nourishment and waste? Do you realize that there is no evidence that icing my damaged tissue is a good thing; that in fact, the opposite is true?"

As my good buddy Joe Smith likes to say in such circumstances, "Game, set, match."

Chapter 8

Do No Additional Harm (Even if that Means Just "Chilling")

Nearly all American physicians take a vow called the "Hippocratic Oath." And, this is not just some passive declaration made at graduation which is promptly forgotten. But instead, this oath is supposed to serve as the driving force behind all clinical decisions made by all physicians who have taken the oath. Indeed, amazingly, this oath has changed little in the thousands of years since it was first proposed.

One of the fundamental principles of this oath is to always strive to "do no harm."

The idea is basic: the physician must decide if doing something is *better* than doing nothing. If there is likely to be more harm than good in any particular intervention, the rule clearly commands physicians not to undertake the intervention.

In most cases, the decision process is rather straightforward. Practicing what is called "evidence based medicine," the physician examines the patient, reviews all available (credible) information regarding the problem, as well as potential interventions, discusses their findings with the patient, and, when appropriate, with their peers, and then considers all of this gathered information in light of their own personal experiences before making a final decision on the best course of action.

At least in the world of musculoskeletal tissue damage, this is usually a pretty simply analysis: does this intervention help or hurt the body's innate healing process.

For example; if an athlete severely sprains their ankle and a physician is considering a "new" treatment option that calls for the patient to do ten "all out" bare-footed forty-yard wind sprints on wet artificial turf four times per day, followed by an order to run up and down icy stadium stairs in flip-flops for ten minutes every other hour, beginning the first day of the injury and continuing until the problem is fully resolved (or the foot falls off, whichever comes first), the physician would evaluate the athlete's ankle, note what the body's innate healing process was doing, review all related credible information, and make a corresponding decision.

In this case, I deliberately created a scenario that would (obviously) *not* result in the physician ordering the intervention, since there is absolutely no credible information to support such an order and the intervention would clearly hurt, not help, the healing process.

But now let's take a look at another, more familiar intervention: icing damaged tissue. Just as with the last example, the physician would evaluate the athlete's ankle, note what the body's innate healing process was doing, and then review all related credible information before making a determination as to the best course of action.

Again, I deliberately created a scenario that should *not* result in the physician ordering the intervention, since there is no credible information to support such an intervention and this action would clearly hurt, not help, the healing process.

Why? Because the use of ice would delay the delivery of needed supplies to the area, disrupt the healing process, delay the evacuation of waste away from the area – likely even cause more waste to congregate in the area – cause additional tissue damage, and mask pain signals that are needed to prevent position-induced damage (e.g. if the patient cannot tell that a particular position is causing pain because of the numbness around their injury area, they will likely remain in that position despite the fact that doing so is actually hurting them).

With regards to this point, consider the following example: an athlete breaks their collarbone. With the injury still seriously hurting, the athlete ices the area, which helps to reduce the pain, and their doctor puts them in a sling, which just happens to be slightly maladjusted.

Since the icing has made the area numb, the athlete does not realize that the sling is forcing the bone to displace along the fracture line. Thus, they do not report the problem and the misalignment goes unchecked.

Predictably, this disrupts the normal healing process and causes unnecessary pain, which leads to even more icing, followed by continued misalignment, and ultimately concluding with a faulty (sub-optimal) fracture repair.

These particular circumstances might sound unlikely, but, the fact is that minor adjustments are often the difference between slow and fast recovery. Indeed, adhering to the body's demands for positioning changes (as well as providing movement when appropriate) is often the key to ensuring optimal healing.

The above example is not, however, hypothetical. In fact, it is what happened to me when I broke my collarbone in January 2013. The only difference in my case was that I was not using ice (or drugs), and thus, when I noticed the discomfort, I immediately reported the issue to my physician. He then promptly adjusted my sling and the pain immediately subsided.

But, since I am the (overly) curious type, I asked him to readjust the sling back to the original position, just so that we could test the effect that it was having.

Sure enough, the pain immediately returned with such potent force that my doctor immediately reset the sling. In case you are wondering, that marked the prompt end of my experimenting!

Oh, and here's the rest of the story. The often-prescribed protocol for such an injury is to initially remain ridiculously still before eventually (way too far down the line) reintroducing movement. And, believe it or not, this is actually a vast improvement from the past, when all "early" movement was the enemy.

Of course, I, as well as my doctor, knew better and, accordingly, we gradually reintroduced (painless) movement almost immediately.

In fact, I was raising my arm above my head at the point when most people with the injury are still doing their best to remain still. And, I was back distance running before most of those people would even have been able to raise their arm parallel to the floor.

But, make no mistake; this was not because I was lucky or special – far from it – it was because I maintained feeling in the area and thus knew what positions that my body was telling me to avoid while it repaired the damage and because I activated my muscles, which helped deliver needed supplies to the area and simultaneously evacuated the accumulating waste, by doing ever-increasing painless – but still stressful – movements beginning almost immediately.

Now, if you're thinking that this whole "no ice" thing doesn't make sense because your doctor – who presumably took the Oath described above – told you to ice your elbow a couple a years ago when you hurt it playing tennis, no problem.

There is a very reasonable and logical explanation. Physicians often change clinical recommendations when new information becomes available and previously accepted methods – perhaps even some that had never proved to be sufficiently credible in the first place – are rejected.

Keep in mind that, not long ago, physicians actually encouraged their patients to remain still for weeks following a musculoskeletal injury. But, when it was discovered that absolute stillness actually caused vastly more harm than good, physicians promptly stopped recommending weeks-long (or even months-long) stillness.

And now today, controlled movement is often introduced within hours of musculoskeletal surgery. In fact, research in the past fifteen years regarding the need to stress (or "load") tissue during the healing process (through muscle activation) has been so overwhelming that it has effectively ended this entire debate.

Of course, as with many things, this does not mean that doctors or their patients always move fast enough in this regard – it just means that some do and that the information is widely available for all to see.

Oh, and remember Vioxx? This drug was, just a few short years ago, at the forefront of many pain relief protocols. In fact, it remains one of the most prescribed pain relief medications in history.

But, one day, it was discovered that the drug actually caused enormously more harm than good – including far too frequently death – and, accordingly, physicians immediately stopped recommending it.

I doubt that you need any more examples, but here is one from the 1950s that I just cannot skip. When I was growing up, almost everyone below the age of fifteen had their tonsils removed, and yet, today, very, very few people have their tonsils removed.

So what happened? It was discovered that tonsils are an important part of the immune system. Indeed, among other things, they produce and release the ever-important T lymphocytes (or T-cells), and thus removing them does more harm than good. Hence, physicians stopped removing them!

In a perfect world, "credible evidence" should be a prerequisite for all protocols, but medicine simply does not always work that way. Sometimes things remain merely because of their continued lore (icing) and other times they are just hastily introduced before *enough* "credible" evidence is produced (Vioxx). Really, what happens is that "credible evidence" is, sometimes, vague and exists in a blurry area.

That is why things are constantly changing and improving – it might not be ideal, but it is just the way things work in a field where the medical responses for many thousands of ailments are simultaneously, constantly being proposed, tested, refined, and rejected. Some protocols – even glaringly bad ones – can simply get lost in the swirl, for a time at least.

In the examples above, information proved (or is proving) to be the catalyst for change. Things that once appeared to make sense were discarded once previously unknown facts were revealed. Indeed, sometimes it just takes a better understanding of the goal.

Let's think about this abstractly for a moment. If you are standing on the side of the road looking at a large nail forced deep into your car tire and you could easily pull it out with the pliers that you have in your trunk. What should you do?

Well, obviously, any thinking person would do nothing.

The reason is simple: although you want your tire restored to its "pre-nail" state as quickly as possible, at this time, there is no doubt that doing *nothing* is a far better idea than doing the *wrong* thing. And, clearly, pulling the nail out on the side of the road is the wrong thing.

Indeed, if you were to pull the nail out, you would invariably do more harm than good – since your tire would go flat!

However, if you had believed that the nail (inflammation) was the problem, you would also have likely believed that pulling it out (icing) was the solution.

Of course, the *real* problem is the hole that the nail made in your tire, not the nail itself. And thus, at this point, the nail is actually *helping* you achieve your larger goal of keeping the air in your tire.

The point here is that when you are trying to decide what to do (or not do) clearly defining and understanding your goal is invaluable.

There are many examples that could be used to illustrate this point, but the nail in the tire story is one that is very easy to visualize and understand.

We all easily get the point because the related principles are common knowledge and any opposing argument would quickly lose momentum – indeed, everyone would witness the tire going flat!

But, just imagine that someone had said, "To avoid losing air after the nail is pulled, simply let all of the air out of the tire *before* you pull the nail out."

This would sure solve the "problem" of the air escaping from the tire as a result of the nail removal, but this "solution" completely ignores – and indeed sabotages – the *actual* goal of keeping the air in the tire.

Of course, this is quite similar to the "goal" of icing to prevent inflammation (like the nail, the *perceived* problem*)*, despite the damage that it does to the *actual* goal of accelerating the healing process to rid the area of the waste (swelling) that is generated by the inflammatory process.

This solution – letting all of the air out of the tire before taking out the nail – makes perfect sense and is essentially indisputable, but only *if* you believe that the core problem here is the escaping air resulting from the nail being pulled out.

Likewise, with icing, many people *mistakenly* believe that swelling is the core problem, and, as such, will do almost anything to try to prevent it. Of course, from the outside, swelling *appears* to be the core problem, but that analysis is badly flawed.

Sure, we all want the "junk" that comprises "swelling" to leave as quickly as possible, but we must also recognize that swelling is an intricate and vital part of the solution.

Indeed, "swelling" is the product of the phase of the inflammatory process that is "cleaning up the mess" and repairing the damaged tissue. And thus, trying to prevent swelling (by preventing the inflammatory process that is causing it) actually sabotages the *actual* goal: healing!

So, what should you do with regards to the nail in the tire? Well, most of us would conclude that the best course of action would be to cautiously drive directly to a reputable service station and have them pull out the nail and immediately put a tire-plug in the hole.

With that, problem solved! The air stays in and the nail is gone.

Both the actual problem (keeping the air in the tire) and the secondary issue (the nail) are entirely solved.

Likewise, with regards to an injury, the only way to achieve the main goal (healing) while also dealing with the secondary issue (ridding the swelling as quickly as possible) is to move, or "activate," the surrounding muscles as much as *safely* possible.

As I explained in detail in chapter five, the healing process is just as easy to understand as the tire example. The body's innate intelligence *automatically* begins the three-phase healing process (e.g. inflammatory, repair, and remodel) almost instantaneously. Meaning, the moment that you get hurt, the healing begins.

Messages are sent system-wide to "announce" tissue damage and summon needed help. Damaged vessels are constricted, sealed and repaired. Surrounding healthy vessels are dilated and have their permeability increased.

Thus, the body is simultaneously *minimizing* blood leakage from the damaged vessels and utilizing surrounding vessels to their fullest potential to provide the needed supplies to the damaged area.

Certain specialized cells are then brought in to destroy and consume all unwanted matter as others begin repairing the damaged tissue and the process of creating new blood vessels. The waste (swelling) is also prepared for removal.

And, remember, *all* of this is done without *any* direction from any conscious thoughts. Indeed, if we were ever forced to do this "manually," we would likely die from a simple sprained ankle.

But, just because this process occurs automatically, *does not* mean that your actions cannot have the effect of either aiding (muscle activation) or hindering (icing) the healing process.

Indeed, your body does need you to consciously contribute a little effort via muscle activation in and/or around the damaged area.

And no, this is *not* a design flaw! Instead, it is a brilliant mechanical action.

Muscle activation not only plays a key role in the delivery and creation of supplies, it is also the primary catalyst of the repair, remodel, and waste removal processes.

Thus, anything that limits or prevents muscle activation – whether the culprit is ice, stillness, or both – invariably inhibits the healing process.

That said, obviously there are times when stillness is temporarily necessary and the "more harm than good" equation is reversed. But, make no mistake; these moments are extremely rare and exceedingly temporary.

For example, here is an instance when the philosophy could be altered to "ice, ice, maybe."

Let's say that you have no choice but to focus exclusively on the present – perhaps you are stranded on a mountain and need to get to base camp to avoid freezing to death.

Your foot is broken and in such pain that walking is not an option unless you use a hunk of ice next to a lake to halt the inflammatory process and prevent additional swelling.

Obviously, dying is more harmful to you than the consequences of increased damage to your foot and thus, in this case, icing would be recommended. Furthermore, it would hardly violate the Hippocratic Oath if your doctor (somehow) ordered you to temporarily ice that injury.

But, other than exceedingly rare circumstances such as this – or those (occasional) moments in the immediate aftermath of an injury when all movement causes additional pain – immediate muscle activation when ordered by your doctor, no matter how slight it might have to be, is always part of the solution.

Anyway, let's go back to the athlete with the severely sprained ankle and consider how the physician would determine if "muscle activation" would do more harm than good.

First, the physician would examine the patient and determine that they had a (very painful) third-degree ankle sprain. Further, they would almost assuredly conclude that the patient's innate healing process was already in full swing, since the internal bleeding had already been stopped, localized blood flow had been increased, and the skin temperature had been elevated.

The physician would also likely note, however, that excess fluid was beginning to accumulate in and around the damaged area (swelling) as a result of inadequate waste removal from the end of the inflammatory process.

Knowing, from many years of medical study and personal experience that the swelling will ultimately exacerbate the situation and that the only way to evacuate the waste is through the lymphatic system – a system that is basically passive and nearly fully reliant upon muscle activation around the vessels to move the waste – the physician would determine that muscle activation would clearly do more good than harm.

Accordingly, the physician would then almost certainly conclude that muscle activation would not only be indicated, but in fact required. The patient would then likely be instructed to immediately begin activating the muscles around their ankle.

The patient would also be informed that, once the "accumulated fluid" was evacuated, they would have less pain, more function, and an easier and less complicated recovery.

The physician would then proceed to provide simple, but detailed instructions, such as, "Never cause pain and activate as much muscle in the general area as possible, as often as possible. Begin by slightly wiggling your toes and lightly contracting your thigh, calf and foot muscles. When possible, begin moving your ankle in all directions, but NEVER cause any pain."

Now, if you're thinking that I deliberately created a scenario that would result in the physician ordering this intervention (muscle activation), you're right.

I am fully aware of the plethora of clinical, physiological, and scientific evidence that supports this particular protocol. I also realize – just as everyone else who has studied this topic during the past several years – that this intervention *easily* passes the "do no harm" test and also passes the "do a lot of good" test with flying colors.

And, perhaps more importantly, I realize that muscle activation demonstrably helps the body's innate healing process, and is, by design, an integral component of the healing process!

But now, let's get back to the "swelling" part of this story.

The fact is that it doesn't take much effort to move waste through the lymphatic system but, depending on the amount of accumulated fluid, as well as its location, and the efficiency of your system, it might take a long time (e.g. up to numerous hours per day for several days, if not weeks) to move it.

Think of it this way. Imagine that 20,000 cars are simultaneously trying to leave the Yankee Stadium parking lot, but only one of the exit gates will open. No matter how many words are yelled or horns are blown, the gate still only allows three cars at a time to leave.

A similar situation occurs with the lymphatic system. The passageways are narrow and only so much can leave at a time. No matter what a person does, this process will still take time – an amount dependent upon how much congestion there is and the efficiency of a person's lymphatic system.

And, manual muscle activation is, of course, not always possible. Indeed, the degree of physical effort necessary to move all of the waste can become enormously tiring (if not downright painful), and, as such, few of us have the stamina to *optimally* self-activate the muscles around our injury site.

And, since many people are either unwilling or unable to undertake this effort, but *still* want their muscles activated so that they can heal as rapidly as possible, many physicians recommend using a powered muscle stimulator.

I have many years of experience with such devices on a wide-range of injuries, as well as general muscle soreness – including with some of our nation's premier athletes – and have enjoyed enormous success across the board.

What these devices do is simple: they effortlessly (and comfortably) activate the muscles in the damaged area without causing fatigue or pain, thereby increasing the flow of nourishment and the evacuation of waste, or "swelling."

Indeed, you can easily control the intensity of the muscle activation – as well as determine which particular muscles to activate. This allows you to not only target the most appropriate muscles, but also work your way from a slight "twitch" all the way up to significant contraction.

I have a plethora of stories in this regard, but, suffice it to say, I *highly* recommend that you and your physician consider this treatment option.

The only thing that I would advise in this regard – in the event that you choose to utilize one of these tools – is that you ensure that the device that you use is cleared by the FDA for the intended use of increasing circulation (e.g. not a TENS machine), and that the company has a clear history of success.

Finally, you might also want to make note that some of these devices are available only by prescription (e.g. for injuries), while others are available without a prescription (e.g. for tired and/or sore muscles). However, the general design, principles, and functions of both of these devices are highly similar.

Chapter 9

Iceless Recovery: Actual Loading
Protocols that Worked!

> *Loading of Healing Bone, Fibrous Tissue, and Muscle:*
> *Implications for Orthopedic Practice:*
>
> *"One of the most important concepts in orthopedics in this century is the understanding that loading accelerates healing of bone, fibrous tissue, and skeletal muscle."*
>
> **Journal of the American Academy of Orthopedic Surgeons,**
> **September/October 1999**
>
> Joseph A. Buckwalter, M.S., M.D., & Alan J. Grodzinsky, Ph.D.

Loading, which is also known as active recovery, is essential to achieving optimal healing of damaged tissue regardless as to whether you are merely tired and/or sore from a scheduled training session or significantly injured from an unplanned collision with an opponent's outstretched leg that has left you upside down and twisted in the middle of a basketball court.

Of course, there are many different quality loading methods – indeed I have personally observed many different preferred flavors of muscle activation (e.g. self-induced isometric contractions, ankle and other joint pumps, stationary bikes, upper body ergometers, anti-gravity treadmills, free weights, elastic bands, selectorized weight machines, manual resistance, body weight, vibration plates, kettlebells, weighted-medicine balls, electric muscle stimulation, etc…) from professional and elite athlete trainers – but the goal and essential components are always the same no matter the philosophical brand that is used to cause enough pain-free stress to sufficiently activate the involved muscles for the desired period of time, but not enough stress to cause fatigue.

Further, it is critical that you keep in mind that this is a recovery technique, not a training technique or competition. Thus, the exclusive objective of this protocol is to facilitate the healing process (e.g. not to enhance performance or set personal records).

In this chapter, I will lay out the methods that I deem to be the easiest and most effective for a myriad of musculoskeletal conditions based on my decades spent training athletes and observing and advising professional trainers and athletes in the training room.

But, with that said, please keep in mind that you should always first consult your doctor before undertaking any healing regimen. Additionally – and this just my no-compromise opinion – make sure that your doctor is "movement-friendly," if not outright iceless, because, if they are not, finding a new doctor may be the best medicine.

Remember, regardless as to whether you are sore and/or tired or injured, the solution is always the same: achieve the largest amount of non-pain inducing muscle activation through slow, controlled movement of/around the damaged tissue that you can as often and as long as is needed (e.g. five to ten hours per day is not uncommon during the initial recovery period when dealing with serious injuries).

So how exactly does loading work? Well, the principle is basic: simply load or "activate" the tired and/or sore muscles (and/or the muscles surrounding injured tissue) to initiate the cascade of events that literally works to protect the area from further damage, prevent or retard disuse atrophy, increase circulation, and, ultimately, heal the damaged tissue.

Essentially, all that you have to do is "activate the system" since your body is already perfectly equipped to "heal thyself."

Achieving the proper amount of loading is part art and part science, but, for the most part, you can just use your common sense to ensure adequate loading (e.g. not too little and not too much) using the general protocol that I describe in this chapter for your particular condition.

It does not matter if you are "recovering" from a serious ankle sprain or a hard chest workout at your favorite Crossfit box, from a broken finger or a sore pitching shoulder, from a hard MMA-style punch to the face that damaged your TMJ joint or "heavy legs" from running the hills, from tennis elbow to arms so tired from paddling in the ocean that you literally cannot comb your hair, the point remains the same: recovery is recovery no matter how complex or how simple the problem or why your tissue is damaged (or for that matter whether it is "positive" damage resulting from intentional training-induced microtrauma or unwanted negative damage resulting from unintentional accident-induced macrotrauma).

The point is that absolute stillness – or worse, combining absolute stillness with ice – inhibits recovery while the correct amount of muscle activation promotes recovery.

Now, let me just state that, while a great deal of complementary scientific information has surfaced since Drs. Buckwalter and Grodzinsky published their revolutionary article, *"Loading of Healing Bone, Fibrous Tissue, and Muscle: Implications for Orthopedic Practice"* in the Journal of the American Academy of Orthopedic Surgeons in 1999 (such as the role of mechanical loading in musculoskeletal development, maintenance, repair, and remodel and loading-induced angiogenesis and the activated muscles' production and release of myokines and PGC1a, which, among other things, ultimately prevents or retards disuse atrophy and directly affects your rate of healing), I do not believe that there is any need to go into further detail regarding that complementary information at this time, especially since the importance of muscle activation (as it relates to this general topic) is thoroughly covered in previous chapters.

However, with that said, there are many easily accessible peer-reviewed journal articles available online if you want to learn more on the topic of loading and its relationship to healing and/or unloading (think space travel) and its relationship to physical degeneration.

As such, this chapter exclusively focuses on *how* to facilitate recovery via muscle activation for many different musculoskeletal conditions (which, in turn, will also help you prevent further decline).

More specifically, this chapter contains actual firsthand recommendations that I have made to members of my elite network. Thus, if you follow this advice – which is based on well-established physiological fact (e.g. not folklore or some "guru's" unsubstantiated self-promoting claim) – you will literally be doing the same thing that many professional and elite athletes did when they had similar issues.

For both clarity and brevity purposes, I have elected not to focus on the degree of tissue damage, per se, since the simple reality is that the foundational protocol is virtually identical regardless as to the severity of the condition.

But, with that said, if you are in fact injured, do not follow this advice until you find an appropriately-licensed doctor (who agrees with the fundamental tenants of this book, or, as my good friend Dr. Nicholas DiNubile has said for more than thirty years, "Ask them if they have joined the *movement* movement") who advises you to do so.

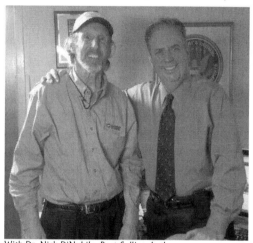

With Dr. Nick DiNubile, Best-Selling Author

Further, even if you are *merely* tired/and or sore but also happen to have an iceless trainer or coach, it can still be very beneficial to discuss these recommendations with them and find the best possible protocol for you.

Now, while such advice is not technically "needed," such related interactions can be extremely helpful if your tiredness and/or soreness is so substantial that the discomfort approaches – if not outright surpasses – the effect of some injuries.

And why do I say this? Well, because I say "merely" with utmost care in this instance. Indeed, many times before I understood exactly what to do I was in a position – as I know many other athletes (maybe even you) have been in as well – where I would gladly have taken a broken finger to the traumatic effects (e.g. punishing prolonged tiredness/soreness) of extreme physical exertion.

For example, I have been so "merely" tired and sore following a hilly marathon that I was unable to walk for nearly a week because of deep, broad muscle soreness in my quads and then proceeded to limp around like a three-legged-dog for another week or so before I could actually claim to be "recovered."

Anyway, regardless as to why you need to activate your muscles, always remember to use your brain and never cause pain. And, also keep in mind, that if you use drugs to mask your pain and/or prevent your innate intelligence from initiating the recovery process – which I personally reject except in the most extreme of circumstances – it becomes virtually impossible to achieve the proper amount of loading and/or optimal healing.

Indeed, if you cannot sufficiently feel the effects of your muscle activation and/or you have pharmacologically turned off your innate intelligence, you may actually cause harm resulting from *too much* or *too little* loading.

As such, if drugs are in your recovery plans, you will want to carefully follow your doctor's orders for healing (which may or may not include loading) rather than solely this advice regarding tissue healing through muscle activation.

Anyway, for the remainder of this chapter, I will be providing specific examples of exactly how to activate your muscles regarding a plethora of related conditions with the same degree of detail that I provide to all members of my elite network – which now includes you!

First, I want to explain some important general information, including a reminder that my idiom – **Use your brain, never cause pain** – is always in play … no exceptions.

And, regardless of what tissue is damaged or where it is located or how it got damaged, the initial goal is to activate the involved muscles with enough pain-free stress to increase circulation (e.g. good stuff in, bad stuff out for the desired period of time) without causing any pain or fatigue.

Always start with extremely minimal effort or movement and only move in pain-free natural planes of movement.

For example, if the condition is in your foot, slightly wiggle your big toe by contracting and relaxing the involved muscles. Only once that feels good should you do the same with your other toes. Once you are able to do that without pain, move your ankle all around and up and down, including ankle pumps, and so on up your leg until you are activating as many muscles as possible in that general area.

If you are unable to activate the muscles in a specific area – perhaps you are wearing a cast or it is simply too painful to activate the specifically-desired muscles or your doctor has instructed you to keep your damaged area still – there is a contingency plan of activating the muscles in the general area that you can employ.

For example, even if you cannot activate the muscles in your foot (e.g. because you are wearing a cast), you can still achieve good results by activating the muscles in your lower and upper leg.

With that said, please note that activating the muscles in your right hand won't help your left foot – obviously.

Why am I recommending that you do this? Well, because as you wiggle your toes by contacting and relaxing the corresponding muscles and then gradually begin to contract and relax the other muscles in that general area; you initiate the cascade of events that ultimately leads to healing.

Additionally, if you fail to provide the needed stress in a timely manner, your repaired tissue will not optimally remodel/form and you will likely develop adhesions and other tissue abnormalities – or what Dr. Nicholas DiNubile calls "unhappy scar tissue" – that will not only complicate and prolong the recovery process, but may also ultimately prevent you from ever regaining one-hundred percent of your pre-damage function and ability.

Thus arises the question that I am often asked: "When is the best time to begin the 'loading' (muscle activation) process?"

My general response is "the sooner the better," but don't get crazy here; clearly there are (rare) times when it is medically necessary to delay the introduction of loading.

But, the good news is, such instances usually call for you to be under direct medical supervision anyway, and so you will almost certainly already have been informed of the need to delay muscle activation (if there is one) by your doctor.

Think about it this way: say, for example, that it is going to snow one inch per hour for the next twenty-four hours. If you go outside and remove the snow every hour on the hour, you will never need more than a stiff broom and minimal effort to keep your sidewalk free and clear of snow.

But, on the other hand, if you wait until the storm is over before you decide to begin clearing the snow, twenty-four inches of frozen white stuff will angrily greet you when you finally open your door, and clearing a path will require a lot more than a broom and casual effort!

Likewise, don't wait until your ankle looks like an overfilled water balloon before you start the activation process – *generally* sooner is better than later.

Now, with all that said, just always keep in mind that you are simply trying to activate your muscles without causing pain or fatigue. At this point, you are not trying to get stronger, build muscle, or do anything else that you would usually deem important when exercising.

Further, note that these are recovery techniques, not training techniques, and, for recovery purposes, they work fabulously well!

If restoring function and/or rebuilding strength are also needed, those missions commence *only* once the damaged tissue is sufficiently healed.

However, with that said, I can assure you that each of those tasks will be much easier if you ensure that the "snow" never accumulates during the healing process (and far less painful).

Further, if you do indeed need to restore function and/or rebuild strength, I strongly recommend the following related guide books: *Becoming a Supple Leopard: The Ultimate Guide to Resolving Pain, Preventing Injury, and Optimizing Athletic Performance* by Dr. Kelly Starrett; and *Framework: Your 7-Step Program for Healthy Muscles, Bones and Joints* by Dr. Nicholas DiNubile.

Powered-Muscle Stimulation

Let me use this opportunity to answer a few of the questions you are likely thinking, such as: do I need a powered-muscle stimulator to optimally recover? If yes, which one is best and do I need a prescription from my doctor?

First of all, you *absolutely DO NOT* need a powered-muscle stimulator to ensure optimal recovery and the reason is simple: muscle activation is muscle activation and healing principles remain the same no matter how that objective is achieved.

However, this technology does make the recovery process easier (sometimes *much* easier), requires much less effort (e.g. essentially none), is often more comfortable, and is faster in many instances.

Additionally, *all* members of my elite network use and recommend the H-Wave® prescription medical device when dealing with injuries (e.g. considerable tissue damage) and the OTC muscle conditioning device, MARC PRO™ for performance and recovery from common exertions

These particular devices are popular within my network because they are effective, easy to use, and feel good. That is all that I will say about them here, but if you want more information, you can easily find related videos of interviews (NOT paid endorsements) that I have recently conducted with numerous trainers of professional and other elite athletes who provide firsthand accounts about their personal usage of these products on the internet (e.g. either H-Wave and MARC PRO company websites or YouTube).

However, with that said, there are several other brands of quality powered-muscle stimulators that I would gladly use if for some reason I was unable to use my preferred brand.

Finally, let me make just one point about those "quality brands." As with many things, there are many more junk products than there are effective products.

Thus, I will give you a quick word of caution: make sure that any medical (e.g. prescription) product that you consider purchasing is cleared by the FDA to increase circulation and prevent or retard disuse atrophy and that any non-injury (e.g. over-the-counter) product is cleared by the FDA to improve or facilitate muscle performance.

You will also want products that are able to contract muscles without simultaneously fatiguing them (e.g., many muscles stimulators designed to tone muscle may be counterproductive in terms of recovery).

Further, I would also advise that you ensure that the manufacturer has published, peer-reviewed evidence validating their indications for use from the FDA.

Now it's time to move on to the protocols for specific musculoskeletal conditions, which, by the way, are all based on my actual experiences with professional and elite athletes.

Further, all muscle activation protocols can be done with or without the aid of a powered-muscle stimulator and related protocols remain the same regardless (the only difference being the placement of muscle-activation pads over the areas of importance when using a powered-muscle stimulator).

Finally, below are some of the most common conditions that I encounter when dealing with athletes of various sports.

This list of protocols is not exhaustive, but should be more than adequate to get the point across for what you need to do for your particular

The examples that I have chosen below represent the cases from my experience that I find to be the most important/common, interesting, and educational.

Note that if you do decide to purchase a powered-muscle stimulator, you will likely find that the manufacturer provides specific protocols for these and many other additional conditions.

Whether you are a CrossFitter, football, basketball, baseball, hockey, soccer, or tennis player, MMA fighter, cyclist, boxer, golfer, runner – heck even a flutist – or whatever else, here we go …

Temporomandibular Joint (TMJ)

My Experiences: I have two very illustrative examples of TMJ conditions. The first was an NFL football player who was hit in the jaw with a helmet (so hard that seeing the replay on TV made *my* jaw hurt) and the second was a professional fighter who was hit in the jaw and literally knocked to the mat from the punch.

In both instances, the athlete had significant pain and greatly restricted motion (e.g. great difficulty opening their mouths).

Further, because of the nature and location of the tissue damage and the general lack of significant muscle density, muscle activation techniques for both athletes were exceedingly difficult – but not impossible – to perform.

The Remedy: *Do no additional harm – no ice!* Once the athletes were each medically cleared to begin assisting their body's natural recovery process, I recommended that each of them undertake gentle isometric contractions of the muscles that control the jaw, followed by more dynamic movement of their jaw once the swelling began to subside.

I recommended that these contractions be done as often as possible during the day without causing pain or fatigue while seated comfortably in a well-padded chair with significant full-body support.

I also reminded the trainers that it is very important to relax all of the muscles in the target area during the activation session.

For this particular condition, a physician-prescribed powered-muscle stimulator makes the job much easier simply because of how long it sometimes takes to achieve the desired amount of muscle activation.

Simply put, the low volume of muscle tissue in this area of the body makes increased circulation and lymphatic drainage slow and time consuming.

Thus, because each of the athletes were under pressurized time constraints to get better and return to their sports, I recommended that each of them use a powered-muscle stimulator to move the process along faster.

If you do not need to accelerate the process, normally both ways work fine, just remember that absolute stillness – *especially* when there is significant damage – is the enemy and time is working against you.

If you decide to use a physician prescribed powered-muscle stimulator, placing the centers of the pads over the TMJ joints will provide good activation once the stimulator is turned on.

That's right, move *both* joints ... moving only one side feels odd and could prove uncomfortable. Besides, it is unlikely that only that one side was damaged even if only one side is painful. However, regardless, simultaneously moving both sides is more comfortable and activating healthy tissue feel's good and does not cause any harm.

In the cases of the two athletes noted above, I recommended three one-hour sessions per day for several days and weaning to zero use once the problem was fully resolved.

NOTE: Use your brain, never cause pain.

Neck, Trapezius (Traps), & Mid-Back

My Experiences: Neck and trap tiredness/soreness is so common among athletes of so many sports that I could literally give dozens of different examples here (seriously, what athlete has never had sore traps?).

However, since the solution is always the same, I will pick my three favorites: (1) an LPGA golfer whose neck and traps were so chronically sore and tired from her grueling training, competition, and travel schedule that it was negatively affecting her swing; (2) a professional cyclist whose traps were so chronically sore that he had literally began changing his riding style, which, in turn, was causing great pain in his hip and low back; and (3) an elite triathlete, whose chronically unrecovered neck and traps were not only affecting his performance, but also his sleep.

The Remedy: *Do no additional harm – no ice!* Since none of these athletes were injured, I recommended to each of them that they begin recovery-based functional movements that involved their tired and sore muscles, such as slowly raising their shoulders to their ears and turning their heads to the right and left and up and down in pain-free natural planes of movement, all while providing slight resistance by tensing their muscles.

Additionally, due to each of their intense training and travel schedules, I also recommended that each assist their body's natural recovery process with an over-the-counter powered-muscle stimulator, with the pads placed on the center of both their right and left traps and just below the lower inside rims of their right and left scapulae, about one inch away from their spines.

Normally, both ways work, but just remember that absolute stillness – *especially* when there is significant damage – is the enemy and time is working against you.

These recommendations – which are, in many ways basic and fundamental – served to (quickly) solve each athlete's condition. And, to this day, they each continue to utilize these tools to combat and prevent chronic tiredness and soreness. Indeed, I was told that the LPGA golfer uses the muscle stimulator every day that she travels or golfs – which is an awful lot of days!

NOTE: Use your brain, never cause pain.

Lower Back

My Experiences: Although I am only going to provide two examples for this section – a professional tennis player and a Winter Olympian – I could easily have picked athletes from virtually any sport, since lower back conditions are universally common and almost always dampen athletic performance – and sometimes outright end careers.

However, since the solution is always the same regardless of what caused the lower back damage, I have picked the two examples that are the easiest to envision.

The first was a top-ranked professional tennis player who had endured lower back pain for basically his entire career, and the second was a world-ranked snowboarder who suffered a bona fide lower back injury.

The tennis player's pain, while substantial, did not prevent him from playing, but certainly minimized his ability to move around the court.

Indeed, the pain never left the forefront of his mind during a match. All that he wanted was relief.

The snowboarder's story, however, was significantly different. He had fully recovered from a lower back injury that he had suffered earlier in his career and was then only seeking to take proactive action to remain healthy.

Further, due to the realities of both of these sports, the athletes' lower backs were constantly abused with their muscles endlessly forced to absorb extreme forces.

Essentially, while their "recovery" goals were vastly different, their protocols were nonetheless identical because it does not matter why or how much tissue is damaged or how severe the tissue damage, since *recovery is recovery.*

The Remedy: *Do no additional harm – no ice!* Only the technically injured athlete needed to get clearance from his doctor before following this advice, but, beyond that, their recovery plans were the same.

I recommended to each of them that they begin recovery-based functional movements that involved the muscles of their lower back, including any and all pain-free natural planes of movement that they were capable of doing, all while providing slight resistance by tensing the related muscles.

I recommended that these contractions be done as often as possible during the day without causing pain or fatigue while seated comfortably in a well-padded chair with full-body support.

I also reminded each of their trainers that it is very important to relax all of the muscles in the target area during the activation session.

Additionally, I recommended that the tennis player assist his body's natural recovery process with a physician-prescribed powered-muscle stimulator and that the Olympian use an over-the-counter powered-muscle stimulator, with the pads placed in the center of both their right and left lower-back muscles about six inches apart (each about one inch from their spines).

Normally, both ways work, but just remember that absolute stillness – *especially* when there is significant damage – is the enemy and time is working against you.

These recommendations – which are, in many ways basic and fundamental – are very powerful and served to solve the related lower-back conditions.

Each of the athlete's trainers has reported to me that the athletes are following this advice and are doing well. One just returned from Wimbledon and the other is awaiting the start of the 2014 Winter Olympics Games.

NOTE: Use your brain, never cause pain.

Shoulders

My Experiences: Although I am going to give you two examples from the MLB in this section, please note that I could have picked athletes from any number of sports that I have worked with, such as tennis, volleyball, or swimming, that require a similar throwing or "throwing-like" motions (regarding the first example) and virtually any athlete (regarding the second example).

However, since the solution is always the same regardless of what caused the shoulder damage, I picked the two most diverse examples to illustrate the point.

The first was an experienced starting MLB pitcher who wanted (needed) a new (effective) recovery regime, and the second was a very well-known member the MLB family who (finally) had his shoulder surgically repaired.

The pitcher's desire was textbook: he simply wanted to recover faster and feel better during the process on a continual basis. The other wanted to recover faster and feel better during the process (I think I see a pattern here), but only for a finite period of time.

Indeed, the only difference between the protocols was that the pitcher's condition took far less time per day to resolve and continued indefinitely while the "MLB family member's" condition required much more time per day, but only lasted a few weeks.

Despite the seemingly great difference between these cases, the protocols were identical because it does not matter why or how much tissue is damaged or how severe the tissue damage, since *recovery is recovery.*

Three seasons have now passed since I first met with the pitcher, and he continues to follow this advice every time that he throws.

In fact, when I recently saw him in the team locker room, he approached me with his hand extended and said, "Gary, I love your machine. I take it everywhere I go and use it every time I throw."

The "MLB family member" also recently told me that, according to his surgeon, his recovery was weeks ahead of schedule and that he feels great. And, more importantly, that he felt really good once he started activating the muscles in the general area.

Indeed, I actually traveled to his house (it was the off season) to provide one-on-one instruction a couple of days post-op and advised him to activate the entire area at least five hours per day and gradually wean to zero use (my estimate was three to five weeks of daily use followed by use as needed).

That said, once he reported to spring training (and his normal work load resumed) he needed to reintroduce his activation schedule periodically for several additional weeks.

The Remedy: *Do no additional harm – no ice!* First off, only the "MLB family member" needed to get clearance from his doctor before following this advice, since the pitcher was not injured.

I recommended to each of them that they begin recovery-based functional movements that involved all of the muscles that moved their affected shoulder, such as slowly raising their shoulder to their ear and rotating their arm in any and all pain-free natural planes of movement that they could, all while providing slight resistance by tensing their muscles.

I also recommended that the pitcher assist his body's natural recovery process with an over-the-counter powered-muscle stimulator and that the "MLB family member" use a physician-prescribed powered-muscle stimulator, with the pads placed on the center of both their right and left traps, just below the lower inside rim of their affected scapula, about one inch away from their spines, and in the middle of the medial and anterior deltoid muscle (e.g. about three inches down from the center top of what most of us call the "upper arm").

Normally, both ways work, but just remember that absolute stillness – *especially* when there is significant damage – is the enemy and time is working against you.

These recommendations – which are, in many ways basic and fundamental – are very powerful and served to (quickly) solve the related shoulder conditions.

Today I estimate that at least twenty MLB pitchers are following the (powered-muscle stimulation) advice that I described above and

another half-dozen or so also use it *before* they throw … very smart!
NOTE: Use your brain, never cause pain.

Upper Arms

My Experiences: For this section, I am going to use the general term "pummeled" to describe the puck, pitch, punch, and pushed conditions of the upper arms described below.

The first was an NHL hockey player who was hit by a puck in the first period of a game (and who, by the way, was amazingly able to return

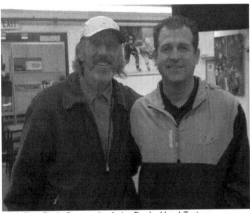

to play in the third period after the trainer followed my recommendations for what to do rather than just sitting there with a bag of ice or taking an early shower).

The second was an MLB player who was hit by a pitch (while, this is an injury that I have provided this same recommendation to

With Tim Clark, Former Anaheim Ducks Head Trainer

countless times, this particular case was slightly different because the player was hit several weeks before I became involved and was having trouble straightening his arm, especially since it was starting to tighten up).

The third was a mixed martial arts (MMA) fighter who suffered a barrage of punches to this area of his arm.

And finally, the fourth was an NBA player who chronically suffered from hits delivered by very large men who were just seeking to establish their "space" on the court – game after game – and frequently used their elbows as battering rams.

Seriously, just imagine your (comparatively much smaller) friends standing next to you in your living room wailing away at your upper arms with their elbows … that would hurt!

Note that in each of these cases the athletes' muscles were sore, not injured, and, as you can see, the line can become a little blurry (indeed, at my age, I think I would call *all* of them injuries if they happened to me!).

The Remedy: *Do no additional harm – no ice!* Since none of these athletes were injured, I recommended to each of them that they (immediately) begin daily functional recovery-based movements on their tired and sore muscles, such as slowly closing and opening their hands (the MMA fighter and NBA player both had conditions on both arms and thus had to make fists and extend out their fingers on both hands) and flexing and releasing all of the muscles in their upper and lower arm in a series of pain-free natural planes of movement, all while providing *slight* resistance by tensing their muscles.

Additionally, due to the fact that the MMA fighter and the NBA player were chronically exposed to this "pummeling," I also recommended that each of them routinely use an over-the-counter powered-muscle stimulator, with the pads placed on the center of both their right and left forearms (palms up) and the middle of the medial and anterior deltoid muscle (e.g. about three inches down from the center top of what most of us call the "upper arm").

Both the NHL and the MLB players also used a powered-muscle stimulator, but only for short-term use to accelerate their recovery process.

Normally, both ways work, but just remember that absolute stillness – *especially* when there is significant damage – is the enemy and time is working against you.

These recommendations served to (quickly) provide relief to each of these athletes; however, such relief was only able to be temporary for the NBA player and MMA fighter given that their respective "pummelings" are not likely to stop anytime soon!

NOTE: Use your brain, never cause pain.

Elbows, Lower Arms, Wrists, Hands, & Fingers

My Experiences: Since conditions to these areas of the body are so common across so many sports, I want to share six different examples with you to make sure that I illustrate this point as clearly as possible.

The first was a professional supercross rider who suffered from (what his trainer) called "arm pump." In short, his forearms would tighten up so much from holding onto his handlebars that he was unable to maintain a solid grip.

And, in his sport, this was a BIG deal, since he would then be unable to optimally control his motorcycle when landing from jumps that often exceeded thirty vertical feet at a very high rate of speed. And, as you can imagine, this became an especially dangerous activity during the final round of a night-long competition.

The second was an accomplished master's level tennis player. He had injured his elbow several years before I had met him and he felt as though his elbow had never really fully recovered.

True, he could still play, but his performance nonetheless persistently suffered, as his elbow would get tired and sore after a just few games, and worse, the soreness would last for several days beyond the match.

His problem actually stemmed from a seemingly minor event – his usage of someone else's racket that had string tension exceeding his strength level – but the problem was anything but minor.

However, despite this frustrating condition, his doctor had discharged him and suggested that he cope with the injury by playing less tennis – the last thing that a devoted tennis player ever wants to hear!

The third was an elite-level rock climber who suffered from chronic soreness in one appendage – from the bend of his elbow to tips of his fingers.

Although still able to climb, his enjoyment of his sport was significantly dampened by this corresponding muscular discomfort and he was forced to forgo some "moves" due to related safety concerns.

The fourth was a professional boxer whose hands would (badly) swell after sparring. Obviously a truly fundamental issue for a boxer, this condition was indeed greatly affecting his training schedule, and a big fight was in his near future!

The fifth was a professional sailor who competed in the America's Cup World Championships. Before I get to his particular condition, I must first touch on this sailor's role on the team.

Indeed, it is true that several sailing positions require IMMENSE physical abilities, but there is one position – the grinder – that get's the crown for most physically challenging.

That was the role of the sailor in this story. His position on the team required him to consistently harness his strength and energy to move the sails in, out, up, and down.

If you have never seen a grinder in action, it is hard to describe the amount of continuous physical work performed. Simply put, the muscles in their fingers, hands, and forearms are pushed to punishing levels of exhaustion.

Seriously, I know of no other sport – except perhaps CrossFit – that places more demand on an athlete's upper body and cardio system simultaneously for such extended periods of time day after day and race after race.

I say all of this to ensure that I explain just how significant the impact was on this grinder's performance – and thus his team's capabilities – when his chronically exhausted forearms would routinely tire and cramp up.

The sixth was a notable flutist. I realize that many musicians are not athletes, but this one was – even if in the slightly abstract sense.

Now, I deliberately saved this one for last just so that I could use the opportunity to reinforce an obvious but often neglected point: it does not matter *why* your muscles are tired and/or sore – heck even yard work counts! – because *recovery is recovery,* period.

Anyway, in this flutist's case, her limiting factor was hand and finger soreness and tiredness resulting from her constant practicing and performing.

By the way, the same point also applied to a hard-rock drummer that I work with who is often soaked with sweat and physically exhausted after an hour (or more) of constant drumming.

In sum, in each of these athletes' (and musicians) cases, I was certain that a properly designed active recovery regime would improve their conditions.

And, since in all of the above examples the athlete had already consulted their physician regarding their "problems" and all were told that there was nothing technically "wrong" with them that rest (read: less activity) wouldn't cure, I was more than happy to help.

This seems like a good time to highlight a novel question to you that I repeatedly ask to to all other members of my elite network: is your problem the result of *overuse* or *under-recovering*?

Based on my personal interactions and observations with so many athletes in so many different sports over such a long period of time, I can tell you that I am CERTAIN that the vast majority of athletes' bodies suffer from *under-recovery*, not the popularly blamed culprit of overuse.

Here's an illustrative example of what I mean. My son – who is an accomplished amateur endurance athlete – told me about a conversation that he recently had at the starting line of a difficult and hilly (26.2-mile) running marathon.

While that distance is certainly a long way by most of our standards – it was mere chump change to the ultra-marathoners who were completing the race to get in some "speed work."

This even caught my son – who is himself an ultramarathoner – off guard. You see, the guys at issue here regularly compete in one-hundred-mile-plus foot races and so, for them, *mere* marathons were a good place to work on their speed.

The point here is incredibly important for all athletes to ingrain in their minds: if your body is chronically *under-recovered*, it will likely *feel* overused REGARDLESS of the amount of work completed.

The Remedy: *Do no additional harm – no ice!* First off, remember, that all of the athletes noted above were medically cleared to begin assisting their body's natural recovery process.

Since they all had basically the same problem – e.g. tired and/or sore muscles in their forearms, hands, and fingers, I recommended to each of them that they (immediately) begin daily functional recovery-based movements on their tired and sore muscles, such as slowly closing and opening their hands, bending and extending their fingers, and flexing and releasing all of the muscles in their lower arms in a series of pain-free natural planes of movement, all while providing slight resistance by tensing their muscles.

I recommended that these contractions be done as often as possible during the day without causing pain or fatigue while seated comfortably in a well-padded chair and with significant full-body support.

I also reminded the trainers that it is very important to relax all of the muscles in the target area during the activation session.

Further, because all of the athletes noted above – save the boxer – often had gaps of time between periods of exertion, I also recommended that they use these recovery techniques *during* practice/competition.

Further, because none of these athletes were at all interested in reducing their commitment to their chosen sports and were likewise not willing to "give up" any of their limited "off-field" time that they didn't have to, I recommended that each of them use an over-the-counter powered-muscle stimulator to move the process along faster.

In fact, I advised the tennis player, grinder, and supercross rider to use the stimulator during "down time," when training, and even when competing (e.g. when sitting on the sideline bench waiting for their next match or race).

But, with that said, normally either way works perfectly fine. Just remember that absolute stillness – *especially* when there is significant damage – is the enemy and time is working against you.

If you decide to use an over-the-counter powered-muscle stimulator, the pad placement for all of the conditions noted above is the same: the center of the affected palm and in the upper-middle of the corresponding forearm (palms up).

In the cases of the six athletes noted above, I recommended thirty to sixty minute (or more when needed) active recovery sessions after any practice or competition.

NOTE: Use your brain, never cause pain.

Ribs

My Experiences: I have two very different examples of this condition. The first was an NFL football player who was hit in the side of his rib cage

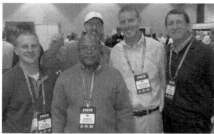

during practice and was questionable for his team's playoff game just three days from then, but who then managed to help his team get the big win, and the other was an elite wind surfer with a cracked rib who was scheduled to attempt to break a world speed record

With all of the Baltimore Ravens trainers

later that week (and ended up achieving his objective!).

If you want to see the rest of this very cool story and enjoy extreme sports, use the search terms "kite surfing record Rob Douglas broken wrist" to find the video on this story and how the wind surfer utilized the protocol that I recommended to his trainer.

Further, here's an interesting side note: before the wind surfer even began his attempt on the world speed record, he knew that he would run out of water (e.g. there was no chance that he could stop in time before crashing!) and yet still went for it! As the video explains, the wind surfer also followed my related advice post-record attempt.

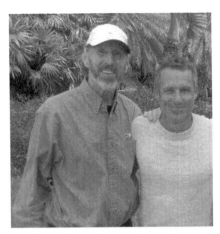

With Mike Gebhardt, Olympic Sailor & elite trainer

Anyway, in both instances, the athletes had significant pain and greatly restricted ranges of motion – including for such simple tasks as taking deep breaths).

Further, because of the nature and location of the tissue damage and the general lack of significant muscle density in the damage areas, muscle activation techniques for both athletes were exceedingly difficult – but not impossible – to perform.

The Remedy: *Do no additional harm – no ice!* Once the athletes were each medically cleared to begin assisting their body's natural recovery process, I recommended that each of them undertake gentle isometric contractions of the muscles that control the rib cage, followed by more dynamic movement of the area once reasonably able.

I recommended that these contractions be done as often as possible during the day without causing pain or fatigue while seated comfortably in a well-padded chair and with significant full-body support. I also reminded the trainers that it is very important to relax all of the muscles in the target area during the activation session.

For this particular condition, a physician-prescribed powered-muscle stimulator makes the job much easier simply because of how long it sometimes takes to achieve the desired amount of muscle activation.

Simply put, the low volume of muscle tissue in this area of the body (and the high degree of associated pain) makes increased circulation and lymphatic drainage slow and time consuming.

Thus, because each of the athletes were under highly pressurized time constraints (e.g. mere days from major moments in their careers) to get better and return to their sports, I recommended that each of them use a powered-muscle stimulator to move the process along faster.

Normally either way works fine, but just remember that absolute stillness – even from these tricky and frustrating conditions – is the enemy and time is working against you.

If you decide to use a physician-prescribed powered-muscle stimulator for your damaged ribs, placing the centers of the pads above and below the damaged tissue in the front AND the back will provide good activation once the stimulator is turned on (I assure you that you will prefer moving both sides of your rib cage at the same time, as moving just one side at a time feels odd and usually uncomfortable). Besides, it is unlikely that only that one side was damaged, even if only one side is painful.

In the cases of the two athletes noted above, I recommended five (or more if needed) one-hour sessions per day for several days and weaning to zero use once the problem was fully resolved.

And, by the way, this same basic protocol would apply to any level of rib area damage (sore and/or tired muscles, bruised ribs, etc.).
NOTE: Use your brain, never cause pain.

Knees, Thighs, Hips, & Glutes

My Experiences: Since conditions to these areas of the body are so common across so many sports, I want to share four different examples with you so that you are ready if/when you suffer from one of these conditions.

The first was a (leading) NBA player who had significant swelling around his knee during the playoffs. Many in the sports media were actually reporting that it was unlikely he would be able to play again that season due to the swelling.

But, I am happy to report that they were wrong and he played (all the way through the team's NBA Finals victory!)

The second athlete was a two-time Olympic track cyclist. Besides the fact that I have never seen bigger, more muscular thighs in my life, I was amazed at his uncanny combination of endurance and power (indeed, I have met athletes with comparable power and others with comparable endurance abilities, but I have never met anyone else with both to this degree, which probably helps explain why he has won more than a dozen national and international titles!).

The third was a professional CrossFitter who was seeking a way to reduce glute soreness. Simply put, his soreness was limiting his training and that was, according to him, unacceptable.

The forth was a NHL player who was battling chronic soreness in the deep muscles that flexed his hips (psoas major and the iliacus muscles).

I say "player" here referring to one particular instance, but I have literally disseminated the same information to at least one-hundred other professional athletes (mostly skaters).

In sum, in each of these athletes' cases, I was certain that a properly designed active recovery regime would improve their conditions.

And, since in all of the above examples the athlete had already consulted their physician regarding their "problem" and all – save the NBA player who was in fact injured at the time but did not require post-season surgery – were told that there was nothing technically "wrong" with them that rest (read: less activity) wouldn't cure, I was more than happy to help.

The Remedy: *Do no additional harm – no ice!* First off, remember, that all of the athletes noted above were medically cleared to begin assisting their body's natural recovery process.

Since only the NBA player and the track cyclist conditions were similar and the CrossFitter and NHL player were not only dissimilar from those two conditions but also dissimilar from each other, there are actually three separate protocols that I must explain here – four if you consider the high volume of activation – which did not include any self-activation – that was needed to get the NBA player back on the court).

I recommended that the NBA player immediately begin activating the muscles in his quads, lower leg, and foot/toes for eight to ten hours per day (or more if needed) using a powered-muscle stimulator, which, once his doctor wrote the Rx for, I provided.

Here, honestly, there simply wasn't time for self-activation and besides, no one could reasonably activate that volume of muscle for that period of time without causing massive systemic fatigue anyway.

Pad placement here was as follows: centers of the pads in the arch of the affected foot (slightly on the inside), behind the knee (slightly to the outside), in the middle of the VMO, and on the lateral quad (about three quarters of the way up the leg).

I recommended that the track cyclist, CrossFitter, and NHL player immediately begin daily functional recovery-based movements on their tired and/or sore muscles, which, for each of them meant the following: (1) the track cyclist: quads, lower leg, and foot/toes; (2) CrossFitter: glutes;

and (3) NHL player: psoas major and the iliacus muscles.

For each of them, I suggested contracting and releasing the muscles in a series of pain-free natural planes of movement, all while providing slight resistance by tensing their muscles.

I recommended that these contractions be done as often as possible during the day without causing pain or fatigue while seated comfortably in a well-padded chair and with significant full-body support.

I also reminded each of their trainers that it is very important to relax all of the muscles in the target area during the activation session.

Further, I recommended that the cyclist, CrossFitter, and NHL player use an over-the-counter powered-muscle stimulator (the NBA player used a physician-prescribed powered-muscle stimulator) to move the process along faster.

But, with that said, normally either way works perfectly fine. Just remember that absolute stillness – *especially* when there is significant damage – is the enemy and time is working against you.

If you decide to use an over-the-counter powered-muscle stimulator the pad placement for the conditions noted above are as follows: (1) the track cyclist's thighs: placing the centers of the pads in the arch of each foot (slightly on the inside), behind the knees (slightly to the outside), in the middle of the VMOs, and on the lateral quads (about three quarters of the way up the leg); (2) the CrossFitter's glutes: placing the centers of the pads in the middle of each glute and on the outer upper glute area; and (3) the NHL player's hip-flexing muscles: placing the centers of the pads over the centers of the central unions of the psoas major and iliacus muscles and over the centers of the piriformis muscle.

In each of these instances, the stimulator provides good activation and helps to solve each of the conditions.

Finally, in the cases of the track cyclist, CrossFitter, and NHL player, I recommended thirty to sixty minute (or more when needed) active recovery sessions after any practice or competition and at least two other sessions per day for at least several weeks (especially for the NHL player). *NOTE: Use your brain, never cause pain.*

Knees, Lower Legs, Ankles, Feet, & Toes

My Experiences: Since conditions to these areas of the body are (again) so common across so many sports, I want to share four different examples with you.

The first was a professional ballet dancer who suffered from sore feet. In short, her feet ALWAYS hurt.

Interestingly, the first time that I met with her and her fellow dancers (about ten of them) I said to them, "Raise your hand if anything hurts."

Quickly, they ALL began to laugh.

They thought I was joking (I was, in fact, not).

Ten seconds or so later, the head therapist said to me, "Gary, everyone here hurts."

Indeed, as the years went by, I learned a great deal about these amazingly tough athletes and realized just how demanding their training truly is.

The second was an elite triathlete who had undergone foot surgery. I knew what he needed to do – e.g. maintain optimal regional circulation and prevent disuse atrophy throughout the entire healing process – and, more importantly, I knew how to do it.

The third was an NFL player who was kicked (HARD!) in the shin. This was actually an unreasonably painful problem (even for an NFL player) and it was significantly restricting his ability to play. And, worse yet, progress (healing) was excruciatingly slow due to inadequate muscle activation prior to my arrival.

By the way, in this instance, the trainers working with this player did not meet me until *after* "time" was not solving the problem. Interestingly, a trainer from another team was actually who recommended me to the player's trainer when he was asked by that trainer if he knew of anything that might help with player's condition.

Anyway, at first, the player's trainer was (understandably) skeptical, asking how exactly I would be able to activate the muscles on the *shin.*

However, once I explained my goal of increasing regional circulation (e.g. good stuff in, bad stuff out) and that I would activate *all* of the muscles in his foot, lower leg, and quads, he immediately agreed that that made sense.

The fourth was an NBA player who was battling chronic foot and calf cramps. The cramps were so severe that he was actually seriously considering retiring from basketball.

I met him because his then-trainer was unable to help him (I did not know that trainer) and so the player actually went back to a trainer that he had worked with from another team (whom I did know).

Anyway, here's the end point: the player did what I and his medical team suggested and he lasted another *six years* in the NBA.

I recommended that the player activate his muscles five hours per day, seven days per week for four to eight weeks after I provided him instruction at his home.

He ended up being so satisfied that, during the remainder of his career, he caused at least two other head trainers to invite me into their training rooms and both now use the product that I taught him to use so many years ago.

Further, the player has personally purchased at least a half-dozen of the over-the-counter version of his medical device and given them to fellow athletes.

This success literally caused at least a dozen other players with similar conditions to follow this advice.

In sum, in each of these athletes' cases, I was certain that a properly designed active recovery regime would improve their conditions.

And, since in all of the above examples the athlete had already consulted their physician regarding their "problems" and all (including the NBA player who was using a physician-prescribed medical product and the triathlete needed to get a prescription from his doctor before he begin activating his muscles) were told that there was nothing technically "wrong" with them that rest (read: less activity) wouldn't cure, I was more than happy to help.

Remember, the triathlete had already had surgery and his problem was *technically* already solved.

The Remedy: *Do no additional harm – no ice!* First off, remember, that all of the athletes noted above were medically cleared to begin assisting their body's natural recovery process.

Since they all had basically the same problem – e.g. tired and/or sore muscles in their lower legs, feet, and/or toes, I recommended to each of them that they (immediately) begin daily functional recovery-based movements on their tired and sore muscles, such as slowly flexing and rotating their ankles, bending and extending their toes, and flexing and releasing all of the muscles in their lower and upper legs in a series of pain-free natural planes of movement, all while providing slight resistance by tensing their muscles.

I recommended that these contractions be done as often as possible during the day without causing pain or fatigue while seated comfortably in a well-padded chair and with significant full-body support. I also reminded the trainers and athletes that it is very important to relax all of the muscles in the target area during the activation session.

Each of them also used an over-the-counter powered-muscle stimulator (save the NBA player and the triathlete who used a medical product) to move the process along faster.

But, with that said, normally either way works perfectly fine. Just remember that absolute stillness – *especially* when there is significant damage – is the enemy and time is working against you.

If you decide to use an over-the-counter powered-muscle stimulator or if your doctor writes an Rx, the pad placement for all of the conditions noted above is the same: placing the centers of the pads in the arch of the affected foot (slightly on the inside), behind the knee (slightly to outside), in the middle of the VMO, and where the top of the foot meets the bottom of the lower leg).

In each of these instances, the stimulator provides good activation and helps to solve each of the conditions.

In the cases of the ballet dancer, football player and triathlete noted above, I recommended thirty to sixty minute (or more when needed) active recovery sessions after any practice or competition and at least three other sessions per day for at least several weeks (especially the triathlete). *NOTE: Use your brain, never cause pain.*

Turf Toe & Hammered Thumb

My Experiences: I know, it seems a bit odd to pair the big toe and the thumb but the fact is that the principles of the two injuries' recovery protocols are very similar. I have two experiences to share with you here.

The first was an NFL football player who injured his toe in a game and had spent a long week and a half hopping around with little to no relief before my advice was sought.

The second was an ex-professional MMA fighter-turned-very successful business man. This story is actually really cool in terms of this book because it served as the inspiration for this chapter.

Here's what happened; I gave a copy of the manuscript for this book to a very accomplished writer and editor whom I knew and asked him to give me feedback.

He then asked me if he could share the book with his colleague (the former MMA fighter) and arrange a conference call at a later date, to which I answered "yes."

Anyway, once on the phone with the editor and the former MMA fighter, the former fighter said, "I get that icing is bad and that you can prove it, but here's my question: I smashed my thumb a few weeks ago and immediately put ice on it. What should I have done instead?"

I then spent the next five minutes explaining what he should have done and why.

Before I knew it, I was writing this comprehensive chapter!

Thanks again to both of you!

Anyway, in both instances, the athlete had significant pain and greatly restricted motion (e.g. couldn't move his big toe and his thumb was stuck in the "straight" position).

Further, because of the nature and location of the tissue damage and the general lack of significant muscle density and compromised circulation, muscle activation techniques for both athletes were a little tricky to perform.

The Remedy: *Do no additional harm – no ice!* Remember, the athlete with the damaged thumb is hypothetical due the fact that my recommendations to him came after the fact. But, with that said, it is the exact same information that I have provided to dozens of others with similar thumb conditions.

Once the NFL player was medically cleared to begin assisting his body's natural recovery process (note: I would have waited for such clearance for the former MMA fighter's thumb injury as well if I had been involved at the time), I recommended that they undertake gentle isometric contractions of the muscles that control the affected foot/lower leg (or hand/forearm for the thumb), followed by more dynamic movement of the affected toe (or thumb) once the swelling began to subside.

I recommended that these contractions be done as often as possible during the day without causing pain or fatigue while seated comfortably in a well-padded chair with significant full-body support.

I also reminded the trainer and retroactively informed the businessman that it is very important to relax all of the muscles in the target area during the activation session.

For these particular conditions, a physician-prescribed powered-muscle stimulator makes the job much easier simply because of how long it sometimes takes to achieve the desired amount of muscle activation.

Simply put, the low volume of muscle tissue in these areas of the body makes increased circulation and lymphatic drainage slow and time consuming, especially when you are trying to move waste out of the big toe since it's such a long way to the "dump!"

Thus, because each of the athletes wanted/would have wanted to resolve their problem as quickly as possible, I recommended that each of them use a physician-prescribed powered-muscle stimulator to move the process along faster.

Normally, both ways work fine, but just remember that absolute stillness – *especially* when there is significant damage – is the enemy and time is working against you.

If you decide to use a physician-prescribed powered-muscle stimulator, placing the centers of the pads in the arch of the affected foot (slightly on the inside), behind the knee (slightly to outside), in the middle of the VMO, and where the top of the foot meets the bottom of the lower leg will provide good activation to help heal the turf toe, and placing the centers of the pads in the in the middle of the palm of the affected hand, the upper-middle of the corresponding forearm (palms up), on the middle of the back of the affected hand, and in the upper-middle of the inside of the upper arm will provide good activation to help heal the thumb.

In the cases of the two athletes noted above, I recommended five one-hour sessions per day for several days and weaning to zero use once the problem was fully resolved.

Following this protocol, the NFL player was walking with little to no pain within a few days and played the following week. And, I am quite confident that the businessman would have preferred to have met me a few weeks sooner!

NOTE: Use your brain, never cause pain.

U.S. Military and Law Enforcement

My Experiences: I added this section not to give loading protocols, but rather to make the appropriate people aware that such protocols do in fact exist.

I have had the honor of working with therapists, trainers, and leaders of some of the most elite individuals in the U.S. Military and various law enforcement agencies.

Conditions have ranged from gunshot wounds to amputations and from general training-related muscle soreness to serious musculoskeletal injuries.

For various reasons, I have decided not to discuss specific cases in the section. However, I do want to invite anyone processing the appropriate credentials (or is/was a member of any such group) who wants to speak with me to feel welcome to contact me via the contact page of garyreinl.com and I would be more than happy to help.

Chapter 10

The University of You: How to Avoid the Cold Shoulder

Welcome to the University of You!

Now that you understand the truth about ice, you probably want to share this information with your family, friends, teammates, coaches, trainers, and/or athletes.

But, you also realize that their general support for icing is deep and widespread, and, as such, it will not be easy to convince many of them without the right conversational approach.

Well, fortunately, I have had thousands of (diverse) conversations on this topic and I have been asked virtually every imaginable question. And, as such, I have heard countless, widely-varying responses and have witnessed the full gamut of facial reactions.

The below questions and answers represent the most common questions that I receive on the topic as well as the best answers for each of them. For me, and hopefully now you, these answers convey what to say to each particular question to ensure that you have the greatest possible effect on your listener.

This chapter is designed to equip you with the tools necessary to provide a university-level educational explanation on the topic of icing damaged tissue. Although it is rich in details, the main purpose of this chapter is to familiarize you with the most common questions/objections that you will likely hear and to provide answers that will enhance your audience's desire to process and absorb the information.

By design, I have already translated the vast majority of the information from "academicese" to common speech. I find it much easier to talk about this topic in this manner and find it especially helpful in the effort to spread the message to the largest possible audience.

If you are ready to become a proud alumnus of the good ole' U of Y… then let's begin!

During the past several years I have had the opportunity to personally speak with many hundreds of people from various backgrounds about icing – including trainers, doctors, therapists, coaches, athletes, friends, and family members.

They, in turn – assuming that each has spoken to at least ten of their peers, patients, teammates, friends, and family members – have spoken to thousands of others about icing.

Additionally, since I readily invite and indeed encourage everyone in my "iceless" network to share their related experiences with me, I have heard literally hundreds of stories about how others have disseminated this information and how their audiences responded.

As a result, I have a very good understanding of what you will need to know to help lead others out of the ice age. I know what questions are most frequently asked and why. And, more importantly, I know the answers to those questions and how to help you find and organize the needed support material.

Indeed, when I began my iceless journey, credible resources to use as support material were very hard to find. True, the ice had already begun to melt, but the general public and both medical and lay reporters (including bloggers) were still mostly in a literary deep freeze. At that time, not a single licensed professional had EVER told me that they outright rejected the ice gurus' dogma.

Fortunately, today a simple internet search like "three phase healing process" will open a stream of information that at least makes this debate two-sided.

But, taking a step back, there is one very interesting point about this that I must first mention. No one that I have ever talked to has ever told me that they had *any* actual evidence whatsoever that icing damaged tissue helped reduce swelling.

Sure, they can point to ice's delaying effect, but nothing about reduction. In retrospect, I find this quite interesting. Additionally, no one has anyone ever claimed to me that they had any firsthand evidence that icing actually *helped* with recovery.

Oddly, most of these same people had long *assumed* that icing helped, but never really considered if it did or not. That was, until some of them were asked by either me or members of my "iceless" network the appropriate questions.

This is likely to be the same for you: what your audience "knows" about icing is based on hearsay – not on any actual field or peer-reviewed evidence – and, as a result, you can quickly expose their own faith in icing to be amazingly shallow.

That said, despite this glaring lack of evidence, no one ever told me that they opposed ice either. That was, until 2011.

The first head trainer to directly declare his feelings regarding the use of ice to me was Keith Dugger, the head trainer of the Colorado Rockies.

The date was January 4, 2011. I had first met Keith in Orlando, Florida, just a few weeks prior at the MLB trainer's annual meeting, but had already made my way to Colorado to see him.

The MLB meeting is among my favorite events, as baseball celebrities populate the hall and ESPN even sets up a studio outside of the hall. Each year, I am fortunate enough to get to talk with many, many people at this event, but in 2010, I was particularly lucky to get to talk with Keith.

I quickly realized that this incredibly humble and polite man was someone whom I especially wanted to work with. After a brief conversation, Keith invited me to come to Denver as soon as possible.

Once there, we talked for about an hour and half and had a very detailed discussion regarding injury prevention and recovery. Remember, this occurred more than twelve months before I published my *"Anti" Inflammatory* article and more than eighteen months before my video interview with Dr. Kelly Starrett was posted online.

At this point, I was a long, long way from possessing the confidence, desire, or, quite frankly, knowledge, to attempt to outright debunk the use the ice.

Nonetheless, Keith did make a few comments during our training room meeting that led me to believe that he was not a big fan of ice. He did not say anything definitive, but I clearly sensed that something was not aligned between him and the ice gurus.

Following a private tour of the complex, he and I stood chatting in the lobby of Coors Stadium.

Then, just as we were about to part, I asked him, "So how do you feel about ice?"

Without hesitation, he replied, "I'm not a believer, I don't use it."

As I walked out of the glass doors of building I was a bit stunned, but also encouraged and perhaps even slightly emboldened.

Out loud, I said to myself, "This is the beginning of the end of the ice age."

I finally heard my view come from the mouth of someone else at the highest level of professional athletics and that was just the spark that I needed. Very soon thereafter, my co-authors and I started writing our *"Anti" Inflammatory* article.

Since my meeting with Keith, many pro trainers have openly stated similar feelings about ice. But still, even today, all these months later, the conventional wisdom about icing is still in transition.

The mass icing epiphany has covered a great many people, but old habits die hard for some. Indeed, while the movement has rapidly encroached into the mainstream of elite athletics, ice still has a place in the eyes of far too many.

But, obviously, showing everyone these facts and providing the corresponding complete explanation is my principal reason for writing this book!

But, believe it or not, some pro trainers actually still regularly use ice despite the overwhelming evidence all around them. And, quite frankly, a few of them would likely find my position on the topic of icing misguided, if not straight-up outrageous, especially those who have never spoken with me directly about icing.

In fact, the following is an example from May 2013, when I was at the annual NBA trainers' meeting in Chicago. This interaction goes to further show just how new this proposition still is in some quarters of professional athletics.

As you will see below, once I laid out the facts, the truth about icing was obvious to the trainer, but, before that, the proposition was clearly never even deliberated.

So what exactly occurred? Well, a head trainer who had never before heard me discuss the use of ice to control swelling caught the tail-end of a conversation that I was having with another head trainer.

The "other" head trainer was someone whom I had known for several years and who had sought my advice on several occasions regarding my recommended treatment protocol for injured players. Thus, he was familiar with several parts of my anti-ice explanation.

His exact words that the "new" trainer caught were, "Roger Caplinger [Director, Medical Operations, Milwaukee Brewers Baseball Club] told me that he has just about stopped using ice altogether, and what he said makes sense to me. I've got three guys post-op right now that I would like to get off ice. Please send me more information."

I accordingly replied, "I will send the information and, come to your facility to further explain."

He then said, "Thank you" before walking away.

As you probably guessed, I frequently work with Roger and all members of his major and minor league training staff.

Anyway, with that, the "new" head trainer approached me and said, "You are not talking about acute, correct?"

I asked, "What do you mean by that?"

He said, "When the player first gets hurt."

I replied, "Once the bleeding stops, which is usually within a few minutes, start moving the waste."

He then said, "But you need to stop the swelling first, right?"

I replied, "Do you want to temporarily delay the swelling or move the related waste? Ice will only delay the inflammatory response, it will not, and fortunately cannot, permanently stop the healing process. 'Extra fluid' (swelling) is a necessary step in that process and ice will not (cannot) help move the swelling in the right direction through the lymphatic system. To the contrary, it often does the opposite."

He then looked at me and said, "Come see me at my training facility in early September, I want to hear more."

As he was walking away, he paused and turned before saying, "I guess I won't need ice anymore."

"Not if you are trying to move waste," I replied.

Also around this time, I was meeting with a longtime friend and ally named Mike Paglia. Mike is a physical therapist and former fully scholarshipped Division 1 swimmer for Northeastern University. Currently, he is a senior manager at a multi-billion dollar therapy company.

As such, Mike has personal ground-level experience with icing from both sides (e.g. patient/therapist) of the clinical relationship, as well as a great understanding of the effects of icing from a managerial perspective.

He has also treated scores of professional, collegiate, and world class athletes during the past two decades and I have personally seen him use ice a few times.

Even though I had stated my views regarding ice to Mike numerous times during the previous several years, I had never questioned his use or asked his opinion until this conversation.

On this day, I asked him, "How often do you use ice and why?"

He replied, "When I went through PT school we were taught to use ice for swelling and pain. I never really thought about it, I just did it. But then, over time, I noticed that whenever I put it [ice] over a swollen area, it was still swollen when I removed the ice.

"Soon I stopped using ice for swelling. Now, I use it occasionally as a 'comfort food.' If my patient wants a little ice at the end of their therapy session because they believe it makes them 'feel' better, I give them a little ice. I know it really doesn't help 'clinically,' but, I feel that a little won't hurt either."

Most people that you will talk to will fall into one of the two categories noted above. The first category includes people like Keith and Mike. They already know that ice is an illusionary treatment option. As such, there is no need to deprogram or convince them of anything.

However, while they obviously already "get it," it is still important to maintain an active line of communication with them. Email them new information that you discover and ask them to do the same.

For me, keeping in frequent contact with most everyone in my iceless network has proved to be a very important tool in my own news-spreading efforts. This way, as I see it at least, everyone in the network will always be optimally equipped to lead others out of the ice age.

The second category consists of people in varying stages of the icing transition, such as the other two trainers noted above. I have learned that, regardless as to whether they are on the verge of changing their icing position or have never even heard a contrary point of view on the matter, it is best not to push information on anyone.

Instead, it is much more helpful to simply ask questions and let them direct the learning process. There is no reason to oversell your position and, for me personally at least, taking it slow has almost always proved to be the best protocol.

After all, it is important to remember just how ingrained icing is in most people's minds – it is, after all, STILL the world's most prevalent injury treatment option!

Anyway, notice how I responded to the "new" head trainer above when he said, "You are not talking about acute correct?"

I asked, "What do you mean by that?"

It is very important to make sure that you understand precisely what the other person is asking. If necessary, don't be afraid to ask them to explain exactly what they mean.

I have found that answering the wrong question can damage your advocacy efforts, and likewise giving what is perceived to be an incoherent response quickly leads to confusion and skepticism. That is why it is so important that you remember to apply *only* the facts to the question that you are being asked.

Once that trainer responded, "When the player first gets hurt," I clearly understood what he wanted to know and responded accordingly.

Notice that I did not minimize or attack his question, nor did I over-answer. With icing, as with most things, nobody likes overzealousness in either of those two forms.

I simply said, "Once the bleeding stops, which is usually within a few minutes, start moving the waste."

This answer did exactly what it needed to: gently, but convincingly, defuse a "user" talking point (bleeding) and clearly state my position.

His next question was, "But you need to stop the swelling first, right?"

This is a very common question that you will almost certainly have to deal with. Here, it is crucial that you do not let your desire to "correct" the questioner's premise translate into an inquisition.

That is why I simply answered with my often-epiphany-inducing question.

When he heard me say, "Do you want to temporarily delay the

swelling or move the related waste?" he was forced to stop and think.

And then, before he could respond I inserted a well-known (and indisputable) physiological fact to keep the discussion focused,

"Ice will only delay the inflammatory response, it will not, and fortunately cannot, permanently stop the healing process. 'Extra fluid' (swelling) is a necessary step in that process and ice will not (cannot) help move the swelling in the right direction through the lymphatic system. To the contrary, it often does the opposite."

This comment will almost certainly keep your audience from taking the discussion in any another (irrelevant) direction. And, when you keep them on track at this point, reasonably-informed people tend to (quickly) take this track straight to the light at the end of the tunnel.

However, reaching this point is not the end. Notice how our conversation ended.

He said "I guess I won't need ice anymore."

He clearly just realized that I led him to something profound, but that did not alter my laser-focus.

In a much toned-down voice, I replied, "Not if you are trying to move waste."

I did not give the slightest indication of gloating and did not ever feel that way. Just as you will likely view your "conversions," I did not view this as a personal victory. Rather, I see such events as joint victories.

I simply want people to have the best information. My goal is not to rally people to my "team," I simply want them to have the best protocol for *their* team. And for you, *their* team might actually be *your* team!

Also, now that your grasp of the facts has allowed you to achieve certainty, you may find that you see those still using ice as utilizing a thoroughly-discredited medical tool.

Indeed, the obviousness may even overwhelm you. But it is important that you never let your desire to help others understand the (urgent) need to rid themselves of this visibly ridiculous tool cause you to become aggressive in your persuasion efforts.

Resist the urge to push this down people's throats. It can be hard, but you need to treat each subsequent person that you talk to just like the first person that you explain this to.

After a while, these facts will probably start to seem painfully rudimentary to you. But, to those people who have just always thought ice to be helpful, these facts do not seem so basic – at least not immediately.

And, always keep in mind that you are just having friendly conversations with like people with whom you are just trying to help.

Even if someone is a hardened "true believer," it's okay!

Since the facts are exclusively on your side, all reasonable people that you talk with will release their blind-faith beliefs once you provide the related information.

Also, it does not matter how someone might have become a "true believer." Whether it was through formal education or was simply "learned," these people always have the same fundamental beliefs. And, as such, the facts will similarly set them all free!

Below is a list of the most common questions that you are likely to be asked and the answers that I have learned are best for each question.

When giving each of these answers, always remember to never stray from the following tandem inquiry, *"Seriously, do you honestly believe that your body's natural inflammatory process is a mistake? Or, that your lymphatic system works better when your muscles are functionally incapacitated."*

These fundamental questions set the tone for all related comments and should ALWAYS serve as your "home base."

Unless your audience is so wedded to their beliefs that they refuse to even listen to any contrary views, you should be able to, at the very least, cause them to doubt what they "know."

While these people are (fortunately) the exception, there are those who inexplicably (and often unintentionally) believe that they can regulate their body's natural response to musculoskeletal tissue damage better than their innate intelligence, by, of all things, making that tissue temporarily cold with an ice cube.

I tend to just walk away after politely thanking members of this exceedingly slow to adapt group (perhaps they still let blood as well?), but, if you have the time and want to be entertained with a fairytale, ask them to explain exactly what changes that they would make to better the body's natural healing process, how they would achieve these changes, and why their way would indeed be better.

The very cringeworthy nature of their response may actually induce them to see a glimmer of "the light," but, even if not, you will still likely be provided with some entertaining pseudo sci-fi theory.

Anyway, here are the University of You's most important questions and answers.

Question 1: Icing damaged tissue will prevent swelling, correct?

Answer: Delay it, yes. Prevent it, no. The body's natural response to tissue damage is to constrict the damaged blood vessels and dilate the surrounding vessels.

The reason the damaged vessel constricts is to limit blood loss and help facilitate the construction of a seal or clot, which, by the way, usually takes less than a few minutes.

The reason the surrounding vessels dilate is to get the needed supplies to the area and begin the clean-up and repair process. When you make the area cold, you delay the process, but, fortunately, you do not stop the process. Once the area warms up, your body's innate intelligence resumes the healing process.

Think of it this way: there's a serious car crash on a major highway and dozens of smashed cars are scattered about. Help is clearly needed and is accordingly sought. Immediately, emergency vehicles and tow trucks are summoned to the crash site, but then, without warning, a giant ice storm freezes everything in place and the emergency vehicles are unable to reach the disabled cars.

Finally, after a frigid fifteen minutes, the storm subsides and things begin to warm up. Movement is now again possible.

Do you believe that the disabled cars are still disabled, or do you believe that they were magically repaired because they were "iced"?

Also, do you believe that the emergency vehicles simply returned to their stations thinking "mission accomplished" after the ice was removed, or do you believe that they still proceeded to the crash site to provide the needed assistance?

Question 2: Icing damaged tissue will remove swelling, correct?

Answer: No, but it may *increase* swelling. "Swelling," or accumulated fluid, is removed via the lymphatic system. The lymphatic system is passive system comprised an estimated 180,000-300,000 miles of one-way vessels that have valves designed to prevent the fluid from moving in the wrong direction.

These valves create a series of tiny chambers. Meaning

that the fluid in the lymphatic vessels moves from chamber to chamber when the vessels are compressed by the muscles that surround them. Remember, lymphatic fluid does not move automatically like the blood, which is automatically moved by the pumping action created by the beating heart.

When the fluid moves, a negative pressure is created in the empty chamber. The negative pressure draws fluid from the area of congestion into the vessel and so on.

Since the "system" is nearly fully reliant upon muscle activation around the vessels to move the "accumulated fluid" (swelling), icing the damaged tissue – which all but prevents meaningful muscle activation – is at best a bad idea and at worst counterproductive with regards to swelling.

Why? Well, because movement of the "swelling" away from the area of congestion and back into general circulation is almost entirely halted. In fact, this is often counterproductive because the icing can actually cause the fluid in the vessels to flow in the *wrong* direction.

Essentially, the "cold" causes the one-way valves to open in the wrong direction, which creates *more* swelling. Additionally, due to the realities of fluid dynamics, cold fluid is harder to move than warm fluid.

Look at it this way, suppose I were to hand you two tubes of tooth paste – one which was normal body temperature and another which was fresh out of the freezer – and told you to squeeze each as hard as you could until both tubes were empty.

Which tube do you think would be harder to empty: the frozen one or the warm one?

How about if you had both frozen and unfrozen bottles of water, which would drain faster if you turned both of them upside down?

Utilizing these visuals, the answers are obvious. Clearly, making tissue cold *does not* enhance movement of accumulated fluid.

But, let's get back to moving that "accumulated fluid" (swelling) via muscle activation around the lymphatic vessels. Picture yourself milking a cow ... backwards. Meaning, you start at the bottom and slowly and methodically move your hands up towards the top.

As the chambers empty, negative pressure builds and the (now) empty chambers act like straws and suck up the "swelling." Essentially, the empty chambers are then able to take in more and more "swelling," thereby eliminating the delays caused by excessive accumulated fluid. This process allows the healing process to proceed unencumbered.

"The lymphatic system is a 'scavenger' system that removes excess fluid, protein molecules, debris, and other matter from the tissue spaces. When fluid enters the terminal lymphatic capillaries, any motion in the tissues that intermittently compresses the lymphatic capillaries propels the lymph forward through the lymphatic system, eventually emptying the lymph back into the circulation."

-Textbook of Medical Physiology 10th Edition, Guyton and Hall

Question 3: I am the team trainer and the players want ice, what do I tell them?

Answer: Start with the truth. Now that you know the facts and how to explain the related information, would you put ice on your own swollen ankle? Of course you wouldn't! Don't be afraid to tell your injured players this very fact.

Look at the person with the swollen ankle or knee who is asking for ice, and say, "Do you want to temporarily delay additional swelling or do you want to move the related waste?"

Take a few minutes to explain the purpose of the extra fluid and why moving the waste is *far* more important than any delay tactics could ever be. They are likely to draw on their own personal injury experience and (eventually) realize the merits of what you are saying.

But, if they still want ice and are determined to use it on their own anyway even after you have given them your best explanation, you have done your duty and should then pivot to providing instruction on how to minimize the related pitfalls of icing.

Question 4: Icing damaged tissue reduces pain, correct?

Answer: Yes, well sort of. No doubt, if you make the damaged tissue cold enough it will temporarily mask the pain. But, icing will not reduce the reason you have pain. Therefore, even though you feel less pain, nothing has really changed.

For example, say you break your collar bone and certain positions really hurt. The important question to consider is *why* those particular positions hurt. The reason is simple: it is likely because you are (inadvertently) pushing the bone out of natural alignment and actually causing *additional* damage.

But then, in an effort to make these particular positions no longer hurt, someone insists that you need to ice the area a couple of times each hour for the first several days. You accept their advice and take the ice.

Thus, for the next several days, whenever a position hurts, you use ice. And, since you don't feel the pain, you believe that you are doing the right thing.

However, this is obviously *not* a good plan for the healing process. The pain is alerting you to the additional damage that is being caused and should prompt you to cease doing whatever you are doing to cause these additional problems.

Similarly, if you twist your ankle and have pain – which is mostly the result of accumulated fluid (swelling) – icing, which does not help move the swelling and might actually cause more swelling, is not a good plan either.

Question 5: What if there is too much swelling?

Answer: First of all, do you honestly believe that your body knows how to clot a broken blood vessel (usually within a few minutes), repair it, and then dissolve the clot when the repair is completed, but mistakenly sends too much fluid to the area?

Seriously, think about that for a minute. Hopefully you agree that your body's innate intelligence is pretty good at regulating the amount of fluid sent to a damaged site and that this process is *not* an arbitrary or chaotic event.

Accordingly, if "too much" fluid does begin to

accumulate (swelling), it's not because your body sent too much fluid. Instead, it's because too little fluid has yet been moved through the lymphatic system.

And, since icing damaged tissue virtually halts (if not reverses) the movement of fluid through the lymphatic system, icing is clearly not helpful in this process.

Question 6: Does icing damaged tissue accelerate healing?

Answer: No. True, there are a couple studies that include a variety of "treatment options" which seem to possibly suggest that maybe when ice is incorporated into a certain combination of treatments the patient outcome appears to potentially improve better than the control group.

Sounds convincing, huh?

Of course, those studies are so shallow and flawed that serious researchers question those conclusions. The bottom line is that after forty years of widespread use, there is no peer-reviewed indisputable evidence that icing damaged tissue improves patient outcomes.

Want proof? Here's the final line of a May 2013 Journal of Strength and Conditioning Research/National Strength and Conditioning Association article entitled, *"Topical cooling (icing) delays recovery from eccentric exercise-induced muscle damage."*

"These data suggest that topical cooling, a commonly used clinical intervention appears to not improve but rather delay recovery from eccentric exercise-induced muscle damage."

And, here's the opening line of a 2012 British Journal of Sports Medicine article entitled, *"Cooling an acute muscle injury: can basic scientific theory translate into the clinical setting?"*

"Ice is commonly used after acute muscle strains but there are no clinical studies of its effectiveness."

Finally, here's the conclusion statement from a February 2008 Journal of Emergency Medicine article entitled, *"Is ice right? Does cryotherapy improve outcome for acute soft tissue injury?"*

"There   is   insufficient   evidence   to   suggest   that

cryotherapy improves clinical outcome in the management of soft tissue injuries."

If you are still unconvinced, there are many other articles with similar findings readily accessible on the internet.

Or if you prefer the more common-sense focused angle, consider this question, "Seriously, do you honestly believe that your body's natural inflammatory process is a mistake? Or that your lymphatic system works better when your muscles as functionally incapacitated."

Question 7: Regarding "icing" damaged tissue, isn't something better than nothing?

Answer: Temporarily masking pain and delaying the healing process is generally not a good idea. With that said, there are a few exceptions.

For example, let's say that you fall and sprain your ankle in the middle of the forest, a full three miles from your cabin. There is no phone service and no one knows where you are. It hurts too much to walk and the rough terrain makes crawling unrealistic.

If you do not move, you will certainly freeze to death by morning. As such, you then decide to gather some snow to put it in a plastic bag before affixing the "ice" to your ankle.

Naturally, this reduces the pain and delays swelling. After an hour of icing, your ankle becomes sufficiently numb that you are able to walk on it – albeit not very well.

Of course, walking on such unstable terrain with that damaged ankle will likely cause additional damage and delaying the healing process will cost you later. But, you nonetheless get to survive. So, icing would be completely reasonable and indeed advisable in this circumstance.

Sure, this is an absurd scenario, but such instances are the only cases where ice could be justifiably recommended. If you care about the *right now* more than you care about every other point in the future, icing can be a viable option, but, other than that, its proper use in medicine is *very* focused and limited.

In sum, if you master these seven questions and answers, you will successfully enlighten nearly everyone that you talk with. And, like any instance where the "facts" need to be replaced by *real* facts and many experts have not yet switched sides, the better that you explain the facts, the faster the information will spread among your network.

And, finally, since there are so comparably few outlets for people to learn of this information, the onus is on each of us to help our family, friends, teammates, coaches, trainers, and athletes understand these fundamental principles of their bodies' injury response so that they do not cause any future harm to themselves or their athletes.

Chapter 11

After the Thaw

I have written this chapter to keep everyone focused on the ultimate goal of *ICED!*

True, this is currently futuristic fiction, but, together, we can ensure that this appears like a factual glimpse though the lens of tomorrow.

We CAN change the world of injury response, and below is what I see the future looking like.

When laid out in this way, this scenario provides me with the necessary perspective to focus on the ultimate goal of spreading this information to everyone – whether involved in athletics or not – and I hope that it will do the same for you.

For the sake of everyone else, let's envision this as reality for the not-too-distant future!

The following is the press release from the Museum of Questionable Medical Devices (yes, an actual museum in 2013) that I will be spending the next decade to make a reality.

"Ten years ago when Gary Reinl released his book *ICED!: The Illusionary Treatment Option*, he predicted that the Museum of Questionable Medical Devices located inside the Science Museum of Minnesota would one day soon feature a display of all known icing 'items' and protocols depicting the history of 'cryotherapy' in sports medicine.

At that time, he promised to personally procure the items, organize the protocols, and, then donate his entire collection to the museum for the "Iceless" exhibit once he had 100,000 people – trainers, coaches, athletes, parents, etc. – in his iceless network.

Well, today the 'Iceless' exhibit finally opened and did so with wide public interest. Young athletes marveled at the 'ancient' tools that their parents used to treat their injuries and older athletes could do little more than laugh, cringe, and shake their heads.

Gary was on site for the opening of the exhibit and was flanked by his two closest allies: Dr. Kelly Starrett and Dr. Nicholas DiNubile.

Fittingly, he wore his trademark hat – which had 'ICED!' embroidered on the front and 'Seriously, do you honestly believe that your body's natural inflammatory process is a mistake?' on the back.

In typical form, Gary remained undeniably true to his reputation as the constant, relentless spreader of anti-icing news.

The 'warm-hearted' trio officially opened the exhibit after 'cutting' the ribbon. But, of course, they could not pass up the chance to dance on icing's watery grave.

Instead of traditional ribbon-cutting, the museum obliged to their request of marking this monumental medical event in Gary's preferred manner: by creating a ribbon out of red, white, and blue colored ice cubes strung together by polyglactin – the material used for dissolvable stitches – and allowing the trio to melt the ribbon using the friction generated from each of them rubbing their hands together.

As the ice and water mixture hit the floor, Gary looked at Dr. Starrett and said, 'The ice age is officially over!'

Relieved and proud of the charge that he led, he looked to the cameras, who were filming a documentary about icing's rapid fall from grace, and said, 'We did it! Trainers, coaches, athletes, doctors, bloggers, and parents all joined together to take down the world's most prevalent injury treatment 'option.'

'Despite near-unanimous support amongst the 'experts,' WE – just a bunch of competent critical-thinkers merely analyzing basic physiological facts – ushered in perhaps the fastest major transition in medical history!

'They told us that 2+2=5 and we said 'no!' Now we heal better and get to get back to doing the sports that we love that much faster!'

These remarks were met by thunderous self-congratulatory cheers from the crowd as the first group of invited guests made their way into the massive room that houses the collection.

As these first visitors – which included more than 150 current and former trainers, athletes, and sports-medicine reporters – got their first glimpses of the showcased items, frequent spurts of laughter quickly ensued as the men and women exchanged their icing 'war' stories.

'Remember those horrible ice baths!' blurted out one former player as another quickly replied, 'OF COURSE! I still have nightmares about them! Those things would be better suited for a medieval torture museum than here!'

One hall-of-fame basketball player even exclaimed that he was 'certain' that his career was extended by 'several years' thanks to the information contained in *ICED!* But, even more telling than this player's words was the fact that numerous other guests simultaneously shook their heads in agreement at the player's proclamation.

One other guest even looked over to the player pointing to the finger that he wears his second championship ring on.

As the player smiled, the guest proceeded to rub his thumb and fingers together alluding to the additional money the player had earned in those final years.

The player then pointed at the guest, now sporting a huge adorning smile, before winking at him.

The player than glanced over at Gary and gave a slight 'thank you' nod before saying, 'But it is my son – who now will never be subjected to these harmful tools – that I am most happy for. It will do untold good for his career – college, and hopefully beyond.'

The President of the museum, Eric Jolly, also proudly announced that the 'Iceless' exhibit is officially the largest collection of cold therapy items in the world, adding that he was thrilled that Gary chose this museum as the final resting place for his vast collection of icing artifacts.

We at the museum had been prepared for serious attention, but even we were surprised by the enormous interest generated by the public. Numerous curators have already inquired about our willingness to loan parts of the collection and countless reporters from all over the country were on hand to cover today's grand opening.

But, perhaps this should not have come as such a surprise. As Gary and his allies have been saying for years, this is one of those exceedingly rare medical issues that affects nearly everyone many times in their lives. After all, who hasn't iced a sore knee?

And, as it has been Gary's mission since day one to spread this news to everyone, we could not be happier to further his mission. For him, this has been a personal calling – as he is a lifelong runner, is the father of a devout runner, and has worked with professional athletes for decades – and we intend to manage this exhibit with that that same level of passion.

Gary could not just sit back and watch elite athletes getting iced – let alone think about the millions of amateur and little league athletes getting iced – without trying to give them this message. We intend to commemorate his success in that effort to the best of our ability.

Although the collection includes a vast and diverse array of items and related support material – including over one-hundred items, three-hundred videos, forty books, more than five-thousand pages of protocols and notes, and thousands of journal articles – perhaps the most intriguing highlight is the display of the first copy of *ICED!*

The book, which has never been opened, sits in a glass case that somehow floats in midair about forty inches above the ground in the center of the room.

As the ever-metaphor-obsessed Gary likes to say when asked how it remains in place, 'Like many things that appear to be something they are not, it's just an illusion – enjoy!'

Immediately to the right of the 'floating book' is a 'wireless' ice bag from 1960s.

This was the first item in Gary's original collection. It looks like a deflated balloon with a three-inch metal screw top. It is rumored that Gary got it as a gift from his longtime friend Gary Vitti, the legendary former head trainer of the Los Angeles Lakers, who was also on hand for today's grand opening.

Neither of them would confirm nor deny the rumor, but, regardless as to where it came from or who might have used it, it is a classic reminder of the past.

Although it can be hard to decide what to look at next, the narrated story board on the back wall was a very popular choice throughout the day.

The narrator (Gary) begins with the following words, 'Believe it or not, nearly everyone once used ice to 'treat' musculoskeletal injuries. I know, it sounds ridiculous now, but, like all of the other items featured here at the Museum of Questionable Medical Devices, all items in the 'Iceless' collection were actually used by real people.

'In fact, since all items in the collection came directly from professional training rooms run by trainers in my iceless network, it is very likely that some of the greatest athletes in modern history actually used these very devices and followed the related protocols.'

The video then goes on to show professional athletes sitting on team benches and training rooms with ice packs strapped to various parts of their bodies.

This 'highlights' reel – which features nearly 100 different players, each for about three seconds – quickly proved to be a favorite of numerous former players who laughed and hit each other's arms as many of them watched themselves and/or their teammates mindlessly freezing their skin.

However, those athletes not featured in the highlights reel need not despair!

The display's attached touchscreen gives simple access to pictures and/or videos of more than 5,000 professional athletes using (now) discredited icing techniques.

This vast collection was compiled to give visitors a clear understanding of just how widespread icing was – indeed far more so than many previously-discredited medical practices!

Visitors are also encouraged to watch interactive videos on a piece of history that we Minnesotans particularly cherish: fifty-five completely refurbished custom box seats from the Metrodome, the Vikings old stadium before it was demolished in 2018.

Each seat even has its own custom viewing screen that rises from the floor once you are seated. All written and video material is easily located via a voice controlled locator system.

For example; if you want to see all videos that involve a player or trainer from the Minnesota Twins, you simply say, video, Twins. If you want to narrow your search, just say, video, Twins, 1980s.

Plus, since all written material is also stored digitally, you can read any article, book, protocol or related notes with ease.

But it gets even better!

You can enjoy this cool modern technology while taking part in the old-time medical practice of icing your leg!

Many of our youngest visitors had never had ice on them and our older patrons loved the nostalgic feel of the cold on their legs.

The armrests of the chairs also serve as coolers and thus, all that visitors need to do to 'treat' themselves with ice is to open up their right armrest and pull out the ice pack.

We suspect that this will be much more popular in the summer than during our Minnesota winter, but it was nonetheless a hit!

And, for our most thrill-seeking visitors, our 'Iceless' exhibit also allows patrons to get even more personally involved.

After signing a waiver, visitors aged fourteen and up can operate the cold air device that blows air so cold that it can literally cause frostbite in less than five minutes.

Indeed, during its active use days, it actually *did* cause frostbite many times! But, for the safety of visitors, this particular machine automatically shuts off after ninety seconds.

But, those too young or unwilling to do this to themselves can still toy with the device. Of course, this is not quite the same as aiming the frigid air towards living tissue, but it is very entertaining nonetheless.

These visitors can get the effect of the once-cripplingly expensive device by utilizing hand controls to blow the air on a lifelike medical model.

As users aim the air on particular parts of the high-tech mannequin's body, the machine digitally displays the surface temperature of the targeted tissue. And, on a screen off to the side, users can watch what happens internally as vessels constrict and try to weather the ice storm.

Many of today's users remained in disbelief that this device was not only legally available, but actually popular just a decade ago.

And, in one final interactive exhibit, patrons – or at least those who brought their bathing suits – can dive into a good old fashion ice bath!

Well, they cannot exactly 'dive' in, as the tub is but ten inches deep, but they can still get the feel of what local Minnesota waters feel like in the wintertime!

Indeed, only about fifteen of today's visitors opted for this highly-interactive display. However, interestingly, today's post-exit surveys indicated that over 94% of the guests were aware of this option prior to coming today.

As Gary told the curator with regards to this phenomenon, 'Interesting, isn't it that the people's collective common sense dictated that even just *sampling* an ice bath was not advisable!'

However, unless over eighteen-years-old and willing to sign a waiver, museum staff required that patrons limit their exposure time in the water to just ninety seconds – a far cry from the long baths athletes of yesteryear endured.

But, of those fifteen brave souls who actually made their way into the water, only six of them made it more than ten seconds and just three of them made it the full ninety seconds (or more).

One young girl was even overheard asking her father, 'If it is too dangerous for me to go in for just a few seconds, why would anyone ever take an ice bath?'

The father was as perplexed by the question as everyone else who heard her ask it.

This was despite the fact that just ten years ago this was deemed not just advisable for many of the world's most elite athletes, but imperative for them to be their best.

The 'toughest' and 'most dedicated' were generally the only ones willing to subject their bodies to this torture, and did so just so that they could gain an 'edge.'

However, as Gary joked to several patrons throughout the day, 'This hardly gave an edge to anyone, just an unwelcome numb and often a chill!

'It was like a mean coach one day made this his punishment for some of his misbehaving players, you know, just to make an example out of them, and somehow, someway, it caught on. Unfortunately, the origination point is probably not at all sinister, but still equally mindless.'

In any event, those patrons who did not seek to torture themselves were still able to get the effect of the ice bath by submerging their arms and hands into the icy water.

Interestingly, however, among this group of unwilling ice bathers were the substantial numbers of current and former players who had actually taken ice baths in the past. Their collective disdain was apparent with their complete shunning of this interactive exhibit.

In fact, a few said that using that modality was the unchallenged low point in their careers.

For the several hundred opening day visitors who chose not to freeze themselves with either the cold air or in the ice bath, the exhibit also offered a much less involved sampling method.

Below the photos of several superstar NFL and MLB players pictured self-administering ice massages using paper cups – as well as the cases that display those very cups – visitors can use similar cups to give themselves ice massages.

And finally, for those really 'hands on' types who like to share their adventures with their friends and family, the exhibit features a 'treatment area' that includes real equipment and supplies.

Of course, icing has now been proven to cause damage in many instances, and, as such, only those who have signed a waiver are permitted to enter.

Visitors can try numerous items and even take advantage of video cameras at each station – which can send video of visitors using each device directly to their phone (free of charge).

In addition, each item has a summary card that describes what the manufacturer claimed that it did, the item's detailed sales history, and a fact-finder that compares the claims to physiological reality. Every piece of support material also clearly states where and when the item was used and a highlights list of who was known to have used it.

Supreme interactivity was the museum's goal and today's visitors all seemed to feel that this goal was more than met in this exhibit!

Furthermore, for die-hard icing buffs, there is a 'parts' bin near the exit that contains parts from more than five-hundred different 'ice age' items.

And, if rummaging through this bizarre collection is not enough, visitors can make one final stop at the 'Ice Grave' – an exceedingly unconventional display that Gary deemed to be of utmost necessity.

This massive container contains tiny smashed pieces – each usually less than the size of a penny – from more than 2,500 icing tools.

Every one of the items had come directly from a pro training room before being ceremoniously cut or crushed into minuscule mementos that every visitor is invited to choose from to remember their visit to the 'Iceless' display at the Museum of Questionable Medical Devices.

The curators warn, however, that icing related tools are becoming harder and harder to come by and accordingly, that the bin probably won't be there forever."

For more information about this or any other displays at the Science Museum of Minnesota, please visit: http://www.smm.org/visit.

Made in the USA
San Bernardino, CA
04 January 2014